Praise for *Lady Doctors*

'An illuminating and inspiring history of six exceptional Indian women determined to endure and defy societal opposition for the sake of the greater good. Breathtaking too is Rao's investigative prowess—the way she interrogates existing misconceptions, draws on hitherto neglected source material, and takes into account not just the traditional norms but colonial oppression and racist attitudes these women had to navigate in their pursuit of medicine.'

— Tiffany Tsao, author of *The Majesties*

'Kavitha Rao's *Lady Doctors* is several things all at once: a richly satisfying read about a set of extraordinary women; a positively enlightening account of how ordinary girls, against the odds and through sheer—even painful—determination, became pathbreakers; and a much-needed reminder that Indian history is as much the story of understated, often forgotten pioneers as it is of our run-of-the-mill heroes. I learnt much from *Lady Doctors*, and drew great joy from its pages.'

—Manu S. Pillai,
author of *False Allies: India's Maharajahs in the Age of Ravi Varma*

Lady Doctors

The Untold Stories of India's First Women in Medicine

Kavitha Rao

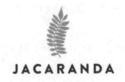

JACARANDA

This edition first published in Great Britain 2023
Jacaranda Books Art Music Ltd
27 Old Gloucester Street,
London WC1N 3AX
www.jacarandabooksartmusic.co.uk

First published by Westland Non-Fiction, an imprint of Westland
Publications Private Limited, in 2021

Image of Dr Anandabai Joshee used with permission from
Drexel University College of Medicine Legacy Center Archives

A CIP catalogue record for this book is available from the British Library

ISBN: 9781914344985
eISBN: 9781914344992

Cover Design: Gavin Morris
Typeset by: Kamillah Brandes
Printed and bound by CPI Group (UK) Ltd, Croydon, CR0 4YY

For Pappa
And all the lady doctors in the family

Contents

Introduction

*'You ask me, why I should do what is not done by any of my sex?
To this I can only say that society has a right to our work as individuals. If anything seems best for all mankind, each one of us
should try to bring it about.'*
— Anandibai Joshi, India's first woman doctor

It was 24 February 1883. A diminutive eighteen-year-old girl stood up
before an entirely male audience in the town hall of Serampore, West
Bengal, seeking approval for an unprecedented plan. Her presence by
itself was worthy of notice. At the time, women did not leave their
homes—certainly not to address men. But what this solemn young
woman was saying was even more unusual. She was announcing her
intention to sail across the ocean, breaking caste rules and courting
ostracism, to study medicine in the US. Alone. The first Indian woman
to ever do so.

The girl was Anandibai Joshi, who would eventually become India's
first woman doctor. On that crucial day, she gave such a convincing
performance that her speech was later turned into a pamphlet. 'Why
do I go to America?' she asked. 'I go to America because I wish to
study medicine. The want of female physicians in India is keenly felt in
every quarter.' Anandibai went on to explain that the restricted freedoms allowed to Hindu women in India, and the harassment she had
faced as she walked to school, made it near impossible for her to study
in India. 'To continue to live as a Hindu and go to school in any part
of India is very difficult.'[1]

The maverick Anandibai was followed by other fearless women. Kadambini Ganguly battled colonialism and defamation as a 'whore' to become India's first practising doctor, all while bringing up eight children. Rukhmabai Raut escaped the marriage she had been forced into as a child by divorcing her husband, unheard of for Hindu women at the time. They made medicine an acceptable profession for women, and later, even a respectable one.

Little is known of these unsung women, commonly called 'lady doctors'. They do not appear in our textbooks or museums, and have been largely left out of Indian history. A crater on Venus is named after Anandibai, but not a single road or school in India. Anandibai and Rukhmabai have had biographies written about them in Marathi (Marathi is the language spoken in the Western Indian state of Maharashtra); Rukhmabai was the subject of a 2017 film by Anant Mahadevan and, in 2019, Sameer Vidwans directed a Marathi film about Anandibai. Nevertheless, these women are hardly household names across India, in the way that Sarojini Naidu or Rani Lakshmibai of Jhansi are.

These pioneers would inspire other women to become doctors, women who would go on to found institutes that shaped modern India. In West Bengal, fiery Haimabati Sen—a mere child of ten when widowed—would overcome huge challenges to follow in Kadambini's footsteps. Chennai's Muthulakshmi Reddy would become a fervent social reformer, abolish the devadasi (a system by which girls were dedicated to the worship of a goddess in a temple for the rest of their lives) system and go on to establish the Adyar Cancer Institute. In the princely state of Travancore, Mary Poonen Lukose would become a royal physician, India's first surgeon general and first woman legislator. None of them would be remembered in any significant way, and some, like Haimabati, would be completely erased from memory.

This erasure has consequences. Men will argue that women have made no contributions to science. The truth is that they were often not

Introduction

allowed to. Those that were allowed to study have been forgotten or their achievements diminished. Thus, a generation was reared on the trope that women made worse scientists than men because they were not ambitious, determined or tough enough. Meanwhile, in reality, a host of ambitious, determined, tough women were storming medical colleges, topping their classes and making scientific advances, which was brushed under the carpet.

Their forgotten lives hold many lessons for modern women. How did they defy the popular idea that women were unfit for medicine? How did they persuade medical colleges to open their doors? What did they do to escape the suffocating bonds of family, caste and society? How did lady doctors go from being called 'whores' to highly respected professionals?

All these women had something in common: they were fighters. And they certainly had plenty to fight. In the 1860s, upper-caste Indian women barely left the house, let alone travelled overseas to study. Educating a girl was considered unnecessary; educating them in the sciences even more so. Amongst Hindus, it was considered unlucky to let girls remain unmarried after the age of ten. Girls would often be married and widowed before they were twelve, then spend the rest of their lives in poverty. Across the world, medical colleges banned women from attending.

They faced intense opposition: religious, caste-based and patriarchal. They were stoned, harassed and jeered at. Some of the most feted men in India—including the beloved freedom fighter Bal Gangadhar Tilak—opposed higher education for women. Brilliant women doctors who won medals at university were forced to give them up because men felt threatened.

It is to uncover their hidden stories that I wrote this book. But it was not as easy as it sounds. Like most women of their time, many of them did not keep diaries or write their autobiographies. The memoirs they did write were not thought worthy of preserving, and were lost or destroyed. Haimabati Sen wrote her autobiography, but it remained hidden for years in an old trunk, because no one thought it worthy of notice, not even her family. Some, like Anandibai Joshi, did write letters, but they were in Marathi, and thus unavailable to many as translations were hard to come by.

Often, the flamboyant husbands of lady doctors monopolised the narrative. While some were supportive, others, like Haimabati's, were feckless drunkards. Anandibai Joshi's domineering and abusive husband, Gopalrao Joshi, was given the credit for her success. Similarly, Kadambini's husband, the prominent Brahmo reformer Dwarkanath Ganguly, was much praised for his encouragement of her ambitions. His extensive writings and letters survive—probably carefully preserved—while hers do not.

By the time of Muthulakshmi Reddy and Mary Poonen Lukose, in the 1920s, women had emerged from the shadows of their husbands. But Indian libraries still carry little or nothing about lady doctors of the time. It is a terrible injustice that the writings of Indian lady doctors are mostly to be found in libraries in the UK and US, and not easy for Indians to access. There are several about whom we know nothing beyond their names.

In most cases, I could not trace the relatives of the doctors I wanted to write about, and those I did had no memories of these pioneering women in their families. Given the shortage of material, I have chosen to focus on those lady doctors about whom some information survives, and who seemed to me to have the most compelling and fascinating stories. Often—given they did not maintain diaries—I had to look for insight in the journals of their friends or contemporaries. It is impossible to list every woman doctor, so I have likely overlooked many. For the purposes of this book, I also focused on women who practised Western medicine. I refer to them by their first names, not out of disrespect, but because Indian women often go by their first names.

With all these caveats, it is my hope that this book brings these shadowy women into the limelight and allows readers a glimpse into the unconventional lives of India's first women doctors—and likely India's first women to work outside the home.

'Lady Doctor': The Origin Of The Phrase

These days, doctors are doctors, men or women. The phrase 'lady doctor' seems old-fashioned, even anachronistic. And yet there was a time when the concept of a female doctor was so bizarre that they were classed separately as 'lady doctors'. The term arose in the 1870s in the UK, when women first began to entertain the idea of becoming doctors.

The first mention of this outlandish beast came in the *British Medical Journal* (BMJ) in April 1870. The journal ran a lead article, where it called the lady doctor a 'traitress to her sex.'[2] Women should be dependent on men, rather than follow their own 'eccentric longings for the will-o-the-wisp pleasures of independence', suggested the BMJ, quite seriously. After this, the term 'lady doctor' gained currency, and as we shall see, there continued to be great hostility towards the idea of women as doctors.

In India, the term was popularised by the controversial Countess of Dufferin Fund, which was set up in 1885 by Hariot Dufferin, the wife of the then viceroy of India, to bring medical care to India. Soon, it was adopted widely, and bandied about by the media.

The 'First' Woman Doctor: The Fight Over Definitions

Who was the first woman doctor? The answer lies in how we define it. Were practitioners of traditional medicine—such as Ayurveda (an alternative medicine system practised in India and Nepal)—doctors? By that definition, there were likely many women medical practitioners before Anandibai Joshi. Among practitioners of Western medicine, which of the many different types of medical degrees counted towards being a doctor? Were diploma-holders doctors, or only full MBBS-or

MD-holders? Were those women who got a degree but did not practise doctors?

This confusion is especially pronounced in the history of Indian
women doctors. Anandibai Joshi was the first Indian woman to get a
Western medical degree, a two-year MD from the Women's Medical
College, Pennsylvania. But sadly, she died before she could practise. Rukhmabai Raut, who had an MD from the London School
of Medicine, is widely and mistakenly believed to be the first Indian
woman doctor to actually practice. But between Rukhmabai and
Anandibai was the mostly forgotten Kadambini Ganguly, who began
practising in Kolkata in 1886, a full nine years before Rukhmabai.
Ganguly had three diplomas in medicine, and no MD. Still, she was
licensed to practise.

Before Rukhmabai was also the little-known Motibai Kapadia, the
first woman graduate of Grant Medical College in Mumbai. Motibai
got a medical degree in 1889, only three years after Anandibai.
Kapadia then spent the next forty years working for the Victoria
Jubilee Hospital in Ahmedabad, but there is very little information
about her. Meanwhile, some historians from south India argue that
Muthulakshmi Reddy, who began practising in 1912, was the first
woman doctor because she was the first to obtain an MBBS.

The fact is that the fight over who the first Indian woman doctor
was and is a pointless one, as all were pioneers. Kadambini Ganguly
may have practised before Rukhmabai, but as a lower-caste woman
who defied Hindu conservatives, Rukhmabai had far more challenges
to overcome. Muthulakshmi Reddy may not have been the first woman
doctor, but she built institutions that remain unequalled. Mary Poonen
Lukose came many years later, but she was the first woman surgeon
general in India. It is hard to pinpoint who came first, and who came
later. In any case, we would do better to focus on the unique lives and
achievements of each doctor who finds mention in this book.

CHAPTER ONE

The Originals

'It is not easy to be a pioneer—but oh, it is fascinating! I would not trade one moment, even the worst moment, for all the riches in the world.'

—Elizabeth Blackwell,
the first woman doctor to qualify in the US

To understand Indian women doctors, one must first understand how women doctors in other countries brought down the walls that excluded them.

Many of these stories come to us as myths and legends, and it is hard to sift fact from fiction. Historians have engaged in a fair bit of detective work to figure out which women were real, and which were merely the product of wishful thinking by those who craved to see women in medicine. All, however, are proof that women were desperate for an entry into medicine, often resorting to incredible strategies to worm their way in. They dressed as men, moved to countries other than their own, studied in foreign languages and spent years navigating and battling the system.

It was not only men who stood in their way. Many prominent women also did not believe that women could be capable doctors. Florence Nightingale, for instance, in a letter to the philosopher John Stuart Mill, wrote that women doctors 'have tried to be men, and only succeeded in being "third rate men".'[3] She was brutally critical about what she considered the poor quality of the first women doctors, and described Elizabeth Blackwell, thus: 'as inferior as a 3rd rate apothecary of thirty years ago'.[4] Harriet Beecher Stowe, the author and anti-slavery activist, told Blackwell people would never consult a woman doctor.

Nevertheless, a gradual, tentative sisterhood emerged. Many of the early women doctors in the US and the UK set up institutions such as the London School of Medicine that educated women from across the world. Others funded and helped women across the world travel to the West for their degrees. Most early women doctors were thus connected across continents, with doctor helping doctor.

Similarly, the Edinburgh Seven, a brave group of women who studied medicine at the University of Edinburgh but were denied their degrees, inspired Kadambini Ganguly so much that she travelled all the way to Edinburgh to get her degree. British women doctors flocked in droves to India, sponsored by the Dufferin Fund, which was set up to bring medical care to Indian women. It is another matter that it would later be savagely criticised for its colonialist methods and its preference for European doctors over Indian doctors.

Merit-Ptah: The First Woman Doctor Who Wasn't?

Beginning in the 1930s, stories began to be circulated about the 'first' woman doctor—an Egyptian woman called Merit-Ptah, who lived around 2700 BC. She was widely described in popular history books as the world's first woman physician, and as a role model for women in science. The usual tribute—a crater on the moon—was dedicated to her. Then, in 2019, a study appeared which argued that Merit-Ptah likely never existed and had been created because of an error by Dr Kate Campbell Mead-Hurd, a respected Canadian doctor.

Dr Mead-Hurd was a fascinating figure in her own right. Born in Quebec in 1867, she was one of the early women students at the Women's Medical College of Pennsylvania, a pioneering institute. She was passionate about unearthing the forgotten history of women doctors, who she felt had been erased. After years of successful practice, she devoted the last years of her life to travelling the world and writing a mammoth series of books on women doctors. Sadly, she died soon after the publication of the first book, and her magnum opus remained incomplete.

Dr Mead-Hurd identified Merit-Ptah in her book as the first woman doctor. Mead-Hurd's source for her story was a picture and a tablet in the tomb of a high priest buried in the Valley of Kings, which referred to his mother as 'Merit-Ptah, the chief physician'. The book described how she lived during the 5th dynasty of Egypt's Old Kingdom—circa 2730 BC.

In November 2019, Jakub Kwiecinski, a medical historian at the University of Colorado's School of Medicine, claimed that there was no proof that Merit-Ptah really existed. He said that Mead-Hurd had confused her with another ancient Egyptian woman healer, Peseshet. She was also discovered through the excavation of her son's tomb. A false door in the tomb of Akhethetep, who lived circa 2400 BC, was covered with carvings depicting his mother as the 'overseer of healer women'. It is unclear if Peseshet was actually a physician or a midwife.

The case of Merit-Ptah indicates how eager women doctors were to find icons and role models to lead the way. As Kwiecinski pointed out, 'Even though Merit-Ptah is not an authentic ancient Egyptian woman healer, she is a very real symbol of the 20th century feminist struggle to write women back into the history books, and to open medicine and STEM to women.'[5]

Agnodice Of Athens: The First Woman Gynaecologist

Imagine being an Athenian woman in the 4th century BC. It was the 'Golden Age' of Athens—but not for a woman. The ideal role model at the time was Penelope, the patient and uncomplaining wife of the Greek hero Odysseus, who spent twenty years waiting for him, weaving on a loom.

As an Athenian woman, you were expected to give birth to and rear children—as many as possible—weave, cook and take care of the house. You were discouraged from leaving your home. There were no contraceptives. If you needed to have an abortion, you would have to go to back-alley abortionists, because it was banned. You would give birth with no pain relief, attended to by a male doctor, and likely die in the process. There were no female midwives, because women were forbidden from the profession on pain of death. It was not always like that. Only about a century before Agnodice was born, mothers were aided by female midwives. But as they became more popular, male doctors began to feel threatened. They started to try and treat women, helped by the advance of Hippocratic medicine. Hippocrates' school barred women and soon, midwifery became punishable by death.

This had terrible consequences: women began to die in childbirth. As writer Nicole Saldarriaga explains, 'Despite the willingness of newly trained men to take over the gynaecological profession, women adamantly refused to let male physicians perform examinations or help with deliveries. This shyness earned women an extremely poor reputation with doctors, who began to see women as stubborn creatures with no interest in their own treatment. Many Hippocratic treatises that survive today describe this problem, though none admit that it could have been avoided if men had not outlawed midwifery.'[6]

Into this ghastly scene strode Agnodice, whose name meant 'chaste' or 'pure before justice' in Greek. She was the daughter of an influential and rich Athenian family. Since it was forbidden for women to be doctors at the time, Agnodice cut off her hair, put on a *chiton* (a robe meant for men) and went to medical school in Alexandria, where no one knew her. She is believed to have studied under Herophilus, one of the early anatomists, who knew a lot about female anatomy.

After her return to Athens, she was walking the streets when she heard the cries of a woman in labour. She rushed to her aid, but the woman refused help from a man, impelling Agnodice to take off her chiton to reveal herself. From then on, it is said, women began to flock to her, and Agnodice became the best kept secret of Athenian matrons.

But her sudden popularity did not go unnoticed among the jealous male doctors. They began circulating rumours that the handsome young doctor was seducing his patients and breaking the Hippocratic oath. The husbands of her women patients were alarmed.

Agnodice was summoned for a trial. Needless to say, the jury was composed of male doctors and the husbands of her women patients. In a fit of desperation, she is reported to have done the unthinkable. 'She lifted up her tunic and showed the court her *pudenda*.'[7]

For this shameless display, she was arrested and sentenced to death. But her loyal patients protested angrily and demonstrated outside the courthouse, shouting slogans against their husbands. Eventually, Agnodice was released, and the law against women physicians was also revoked.

Or, so goes the thrilling tale. The truth is we have no evidence that Agnodice existed. Many historians believe she was a mythical figure. Her name, they say, is a dead giveaway, because mythical figures were often given the names of character traits. Her pulling her skirts up is also a well-known gesture in comedy, with many such figures appearing in Greek myth. Nevertheless, Agnodice became a figurehead for women in medicine, and was still used centuries later as an example that demonstrated the importance of midwives and women doctors.

Dr James Barry:
The Macho Surgeon Who Was Born A Woman

In the mid-19th century, Dr James Miranda Barry was one of Britain's most famous surgeons. The brusque military doctor was known for his foul temper, but also admired for his extensive work across the British Empire. In the Crimea, he made an enemy of Florence Nightingale, who described him as 'the most hardened creature I ever met, a brute and a blackguard'.[8] Others who had met the doctor described him as a flirt and 'lady killer'.

In 1865, when Barry died, it was discovered that 'he' was a woman. A woman with stretch marks indicating childbirth, which were noticed by the charwoman who prepared him for burial.

Why did Barry have to live such an elaborate lie?

He was born Margaret Ann Bulkley, to a poor, single mother in Ireland, Mary Ann Bulkley, probably in 1792. At the time, women were forbidden from entering medical school. Barry had no choice but to pretend to be a man.

It was a very successful subterfuge. Barry tricked the University of Edinburgh, the British Army and the Royal College of Surgeons, to arguably become Britain's first female doctor. 'Barry's enrolment as a student in December 1809 marked the start of one of the longest deceptions of gender identity ever recorded, a subterfuge that was to last for 56 years,' writes biographer Michael Du Preez.[9] It would be another fifty years before women were officially admitted to medical schools.

When Barry entered the University of Edinburgh, he pretended to be younger than he was, to explain his hairlessness and small frame.[i] Barry was helped in this plot by his uncle, the painter James Barry, and later by his uncle's influential and liberal circle of friends.

Barry was supremely successful. He would be posted to India, Cape Town and Canada, and carry out the first caesarean operation in Africa, in 1826.

He had what could kindly be described as an eccentric personality. 'He was a vegetarian, kept a goat nearby to drink its milk, carried a small dog named Psyche, and was almost always seen with a trusted servant, Danzer, who would stay by Barry's side for 50 years. Each

---

i   I refer to James Barry with masculine pronouns, as this was how Barry referred to himself throughout his life.

morning, Danzer laid out six small towels for Barry to wrap and conceal his curves and broaden his shoulders.'[10]

Despite his squeaky voice and stacked heels—intended to compensate for his barely five-foot frame—Barry carried off his masculine persona, perhaps because no one could have imagined that a woman would have the courage to pretend to be a man.

There was always gossip, though. In his time in South Africa, an inquiry was launched after a poster was put up accusing Lord Charles Somerset, the governor of the Cape Colony, of 'buggering Dr Barry'. The allegations were never verified, but rumours continued that they had had an affair, and that Somerset knew Barry was a woman.

These days, biographers feud over whether Barry was a transgender person, and if he should be referred to as a man, since he apparently identified as one. Jeremy Dronfield, Barry's biographer, weighed in thus, 'Whether Barry qualifies as transgender in modern terms is complicated. When Margaret became James, it wasn't primarily because she wanted to be a man. She wanted to live the kind of life which in 1809 was impossible for a woman. If Margaret had been born in 1989 instead of 1789, free to be a surgeon and soldier, would she have chosen to become a man? On balance, I don't think so, but Margaret might have identified as non-binary.'[11]

The doctor who signed Barry's death certificate upon his death in 1865 said it was 'none of my business' whether Barry was male or female. The gender-bending Dr Barry lies buried in Kensal Green Cemetery in London.

Dr Elizabeth Blackwell: The First Woman Doctor?

At around the same time James Barry was on his deathbed—pretending to the last—a woman doctor in a different country was trying to find clients for her hard-won skills. Her patients were reluctant but she would persevere.

This woman was Elizabeth Blackwell, British by birth and the first woman in the United States to earn a medical degree, which by some accounts makes her the first woman doctor. *The Lancet* called her the 'first woman medical graduate in the modern meaning of the term'.[12] She would be rejected by twenty-nine medical schools and then finally accepted by the thirtieth, as a joke. A more determined and tenacious woman would be hard to find.

Elizabeth was born in Bristol in 1821 to Hannah and Samuel Blackwell, the fourth of eleven children. Her parents were strict Methodists, but also fervent social reformers. Samuel Blackwell, in particular, was unusual for his time, believing in equality for women, rights for slaves and educational reform. He was a prosperous sugar trader but wrestled with the painful contradiction that most of the sugar in those days was picked by African slaves. Eventually, the Blackwell children would give up eating sugar.

In 1832, the Blackwell family sailed for the New World, prompted by Samuel's desire to bring up his children free of tradition and conservatism. There, Samuel became an out-and-out abolitionist, as did the whole family, a dangerous thing to do in the New York of that time.

Soon the family fortunes deteriorated. Samuel's business failed as an economic depression began to bite. In 1838, Samuel died, leaving the family only 20 dollars to live on, with the youngest Blackwell child being only six. The responsibility of supporting the family fell on the elder Blackwell children, all women, in an era where there were few jobs open to women. The five Blackwell sisters began a school, the only option available to women at the time. Elizabeth was barely seventeen, and was already condemned to teaching twelve-hour days to keep the family afloat.

In the years to follow, Elizabeth would teach, read, write and mingle in intellectual circles. One of her friends was Harriet Beecher Stowe, who would go on to write the anti-slavery book *Uncle Tom's Cabin*. By this time, two of the Blackwell brothers would find jobs, leaving her with more leisure time.

The turning point for her came as she was nursing a dying friend, afflicted with a terrible and painful disease; cancer of the uterus. The friend suggested that Elizabeth study medicine, arguing that if she could have been treated by a lady doctor, she would have been spared such suffering. The Victorian modesty of the time prevented women from seeing male doctors for such ailments. As Elizabeth's biographer Nancy Kline explains, 'Cancer of the uterus was a particularly difficult disease for women of her class and generation, who had been taught to be ashamed of their anatomy and kept profoundly ignorant of how it worked. They were routinely taught to hide their physical selves from men; Victorian modesty dictated that they must.'

If women did go to doctors, they were usually examined and treated behind curtains, which often had terrible consequences. As Kline continues, 'Yet when these women got so sick that they must seek out medical attention, they were forced to go to male doctors, or die unattended. Many of them chose the latter course.'[13]

Initially, Elizabeth was shocked by the suggestion. She had always thought of herself as someone interested in moral and spiritual issues, not the grittiness of the human body. In 1845, there was no anaesthesia and patients endured surgery fully conscious, often kicking and screaming. Doctors did not wash their hands or their instruments before they operated and wore the same coat at every operation. 'The more caked it got with old blood, the more respected and feared they were as surgeons.'[14] Elizabeth, nicknamed 'Miss Shy' by her family, was quiet, retiring, and modest, all qualities that would not equip her for the rough-and-ready medicine of the time.

She had a suitor at the time, but she was determined not to marry, because she thought men would restrict her freedom to find her own path. Eventually, she rejected him and decided to pursue medicine.

Her close friends and relatives reacted with disbelief. Even the very liberal Harriet Beecher Stowe discouraged her from what she thought an impractical scheme. Stowe pointed out that Elizabeth would most likely not get into medical school, and if she did, it would be very expensive. And if she did manage to graduate, no patient would come to a lady doctor, she said.[15]

But the sceptics only strengthened Elizabeth's resolve. She began to write to medical schools, all of which rejected her. In 1845, women were admitted only to 'sectarian' schools that taught alternative medicine, such as homeopathy or hydropathy, considered gentler forms of medicine better suited to women. But Elizabeth did not want to be on the margins of medicine; she wanted to be in the mainstream, even if it meant sawing into bloody, thrashing bodies.

At the time, it cost 3,000 dollars to study medicine. Elizabeth signed up for another teaching position in North Carolina to earn what she needed. She used the time to study medical textbooks and talk with doctors, to find a way into the profession. In 1846, Elizabeth moved to Philadelphia, where she 'shadowed' a couple of eminent doctors, attending lectures and studying anatomy while they tried to help her enter a medical school.

But all her enquiries were met with scorn. While a few doctors helped her, most were amazed at the idea that a woman might try to learn medicine. It was suggested that she disguise herself as a man and study in Paris, but Elizabeth did not want to arrive at her goal by subterfuge. She believed she had every right to study medicine, which she called a 'moral crusade', and she wanted to do it in full public view.

By mid-1846, twenty-nine schools on the East Coast had turned her down. She was now twenty-five—an age by which most women of her class were married and had numerous children—and she began to fear that time was running out. Then, on 20 October 1847, she got a letter from the dean of Geneva Medical College in upstate New York. The letter informed her that the students of the college had considered her proposal and voted her in.

'Resolved that a radical principle of a Republican government is the universal education of both sexes, that to every branch of scientific education the door should be open equally to all, that the application of Elizabeth Blackwell to become a member of our class meets our entire approbation, and in extending our unanimous invitation, we pledge ourselves that no conduct of ours shall cause her to regret her attendance at this institution.'[16]

Elizabeth was delighted. Immediately, she packed and left for Geneva. There, however, she was to receive a rude shock—her acceptance was a farce. The students of the college were a bunch of high-spirited and rowdy local boys who had thought her application to be a hoax. The dean, not wanting to offend Elizabeth's influential sponsor, a local doctor, had gone along with it. When the boys voted to let her in, he was shocked, but did not expect her to actually join.

Thus it was that Elizabeth arrived, dressed in quiet Quaker grey, to a class that was most taken aback to see her. The dean was astonished, and there was total silence in the class as the boys turned to get a glimpse of her. But Elizabeth, with her passel of brothers, was used to rowdy boys.

Over the next few days, Elizabeth was an object of curiosity. She maintained a stiff upper lip, dignified and serious as she had always been, ignoring the notes thrown at her, the hissed comments and the constant stares thrown her way in the town of Geneva. On one occasion, the townsfolk arrived in the class to take a look at her, much to her embarrassment.

Her godsend was the professor of anatomy, Dr James Webster, whom she referred to as 'a fat little fairy in the shape of the professor of anatomy'.[17] Soon, the newspapers got wind of the fact that there was a woman studying medicine along with men. The articles were uniformly patronising. She was described in the *Boston Medical and Surgical Journal* as a pretty little specimen of the feminine gender, and *The Baltimore Sun* wrote that it hoped she would confine her practice to 'diseases of the heart'.[18]

In November 1847, Elizabeth came up against what she called

a 'terrible ordeal': Dr Webster's class finally began to discuss the reproductive system. Webster had a reputation for naughty jokes and profanity. On the first day, Elizabeth wrote, 'I had to pinch my hand till the blood nearly came, and call on Christ to help me from smiling, for that would have ruined everything.'[19] Webster suggested that she study the unit separately.

By this time, Elizabeth had already embarked on a bizarre endeavour: stopping herself from blushing like a Victorian maiden. She believed—such was the state of science at the time—that if she decreased the amount of blood in her body she would not blush as easily, and so she fasted for weeks on end. Nevertheless, she wanted to attend the class. She wrote a compelling letter to Dr Webster. His position, she wrote, might be 'embarrassing when viewed from the low standpoint of impure and unchaste sentiments'. But she was a serious student, for whom anatomy 'excited profound reverence', and she was sure that he too, as a medical man, had been elevated and purified by the study of anatomy. She offered to sit in the back row and take off her bonnet to keep a low profile, if she made him uncomfortable.[20]

Dr Webster was bowled over by the letter. He read it out in class, and then welcomed Elizabeth in, to cheers. After this incident, Elizabeth was treated as one of the boys, and the class in its turn behaved impeccably. She spoke warmly of how men and women could be comrades and equals in ideal circumstances. Nevertheless, the burden of being a pioneer was hers to carry.

On 23 January 1849, Elizabeth graduated. She was twenty-eight. The president of the college called her up, addressing her as Domina (mistress) instead of Domine (master). Elizabeth replied, 'Sir, I thank you; by the help of the Most High it shall be the effort of my life to shed honour upon your diploma.'

But while she had gained the respect of her peers at college, in the real world there was no job to be found for her. American hospitals would not accept women doctors at the time. So, she set sail for Paris, where they were reported to be more accepting of women doctors, with a stopover in England en route.

Punch magazine wrote a poem in her honour:

> Young ladies all, of every clime,
> Especially of Britain,
> Who wholly occupy your time
> In novels or in knitting,
> Whose highest skill is to but to play,
> Sing, dance of French to clack well,
> Reflect on the example, pray,
> Of excellent Miss Blackwell![21]

In England, Elizabeth was showered with praise and invited to party after party; yet, she found that people were not willing to accept a lady physician. She was a novelty at best and deeply dangerous at worst. Even upon her arrival in Paris, she would find herself met with resistance. Eventually, she decided to work at La Maternité, a government-run maternity hospital, where she was placed alongside raw midwives, ten years younger and with scarcely any education. Her years spent getting a degree seemed wasted. But at least she was getting experience.

Elizabeth would deliver babies for twelve hours at a time. She had to learn French, and then learn medical terms. At night, she shared a dormitory with eleven giggling, rambunctious girls. There was also the hint of romance. She was close to a young resident, Hippolyte Blot, a few years her junior.

But then came a terrible setback for Elizabeth. On 4 November 1849, as Elizabeth was ministering to a young infant with an eye infection, a bit of liquid splashed into her eye. She was clocking in a twelve-hour shift, and so wiped it away in her impatience. By the next morning, she could not open her eye. Hippolyte examined her and ordered immediate treatment. Her eye was infected and the infection was spreading to the other eye.

These days, Elizabeth would have been given antibiotics. In 1849, leeches were attached to her forehead. She was purged, wrapped in mustard plasters and cold compresses were placed over her eyes. Hippolyte had to remove the film developing over her eyes every few hours.

After three days of this, the dreadful truth dawned on Elizabeth. She was blind in her left eye. She lay in the dark, wondering if her entire career was over. Her right eye gradually cleared, but the left remained blind. The incident destroyed her budding romance and her dream of being a surgeon.

In August 1850, her eye was removed and a glass eye put in its place. It was the death of a glorious dream. She could now never be a surgeon. But valiantly, she pushed on. She could still be a doctor.

By the end of 1850, Elizabeth went back to London, determined to get more experience. There she met a young woman who desperately wanted to become a nurse, but was thwarted by her parents: one Florence Nightingale. Florence had her own radical ideas about hygiene, not shared by many at the time. Florence believed that dirt, drink, diet, dampness, draughts and drains caused diseases, at a time when doctors did not even wash their hands before amputating. Elizabeth would go on to share that view, and become a huge advocate of good medical hygiene.

While friends initially, their paths soon diverged. Nightingale took pains to disguise her opinion of Elizabeth, but she secretly despised her. In fact, Nightingale was fundamentally against women doctors, believing that they were all second-rate, and would be better off being good nurses instead. In 1860, in her book *Notes on Nursing*, she would savagely criticise pioneers like Elizabeth who sought to be doctors. She urged them to avoid the popular 'jargon' of the time: 'namely, about the "rights" of women, which urges women to do all that men do, including the medical and other professions, merely because men do it, and without regard to whether this is the best that women can do'. Nightingale argued, 'You do not want the effect of your good things to be, "How wonderful for a woman!"'[22]

Regardless of what Nightingale and other British women in related professions thought, Elizabeth pressed ahead. By this time, she had come to the conclusion that New York would offer the best opportunities for a lady doctor. She returned to the US and looked for a room to rent in New York, but was turned away time and time again. In those days, female physicians were thought to be abortionists, and thus shunned. When she eventually found a room to rent, no patients came. So, the resourceful Elizabeth found another route to make her way into the community: delivering lectures on women's health. She launched a series of lectures, which would later be published under the unwieldy title *The Laws of Life with Special Reference to the Education of Girls*.

The ideas she expounded on in the lectures were unusual. Girls should be encouraged to run, climb, ride and dance, said Elizabeth. They should be taught about the working of their own bodies. The audience, mostly Quaker women, were enthralled by her ideas. Soon, patients began to come, at first mostly women and children, and then, eventually, men.

Between 1854 and 1874, Elizabeth was incredibly busy, setting up all kinds of pioneering institutions. In these twenty years, she went further than any other woman doctor. She would travel back and forth across the Atlantic, working to bring more women into medicine in both the US and the UK.

In 1854, she opened the New York Dispensary for Poor Women and Children in one of the city's poorest wards, the Eleventh Ward, where people often lived ten to a room. So filthy were the surroundings that pigs ran in the streets and blood from nearby slaughterhouses flowed freely. In this foetid atmosphere, Elizabeth became a tireless advocate for public health. By then, her sister, Emily Blackwell, had also graduated as a doctor.

Subsequently, in 1859, Elizabeth became the first woman doctor to be registered in the British Medical Registry. This was a massive triumph, one that would later influence a whole generation of British women.

The Blackwell sisters were in the process of starting an all-women's medical school when the American Civil War began. The Blackwells had always been fervent abolitionists right from their youth. They immediately threw themselves into the training of women nurses for the wounded. In those days, the army used only male nurses, or at a pinch, untrained and clumsy soldiers. Despite Florence Nightingale's success and fame, the profession of nursing was still thought of as unsuitable for ladies of high birth.

But the Civil War blew these notions out of the water. Nurses, of any sex, were needed—fast. Despite their eagerness to be involved, though, lady doctors were still not accepted. The two sisters never saw the front, and were forced to help from New York, where they trained the nurses. But the Civil War made the Blackwells realise the need for improving sanitation and prompted a lifelong interest in hygiene and handwashing. Soldiers were treated in such unsanitary conditions that they often died of infection rather than their wounds, or of diseases such as typhus or dysentery.

When the war finally limped to an end in 1865, the Blackwells were all the more convinced of the need for an all-women's college. In 1868, the Women's Medical College was set up. Elizabeth appointed herself professor of hygiene, a position unique to her medical school. The students were expected to be better than men; they would study medicine for three years—later increased to four—rather than the usual two. They would do clinical work based on a sound knowledge of medicine, and not merely, as Elizabeth put it, dispense 'sympathy'.

The Blackwells' school inspired followers. In 1874, the London

School of Medicine for Women was started by Elizabeth's former student, Sophia Jex-Blake. Elizabeth would teach there, but she butted heads with the formidable Jex-Blake, who had her own ideas of how to do things. Elizabeth finally retired to the English countryside where she wrote several books and articles, mentored young women doctors and campaigned for better hygiene. She would die peacefully at home in 1910, single and independent to the end.

Elizabeth Garrett Anderson: The First British Woman Doctor

Elizabeth Blackwell's success had a ripple effect, particularly across the Atlantic. One young woman in Britain read about Blackwell's achievements and began thinking up strategies to follow in her footsteps.

Elizabeth Garret Anderson, like her namesake, had to overcome daunting prejudice. She was born in Whitechapel in east London, one of the twelve children of pawnbroker Newson Garrett. Like Blackwell's father, Garrett was a liberal man who believed in the education of women.

Elizabeth and her sisters met many early feminists, and were surrounded by career women. Then, purely by chance, she met Elizabeth Blackwell on one of her many trips to Britain in 1859. After that momentous meeting, she decided to become a doctor. One small step for Elizabeth Garret Anderson, but a giant step for women doctors. It was mainly through her efforts that the profession would first be opened up to women in the UK, and then later to Indian women.

But in the early days, Elizabeth found the door constantly slammed in her face. She spent six months as a nurse at Middlesex Hospital, but the male students refused to allow her to attend the medical school to train as a doctor. Undeterred, she employed a private tutor. Eventually, resentful men kicked her out of the hospital as well. She then applied to Oxford, Cambridge, the University of Edinburgh and other top medical schools. All of them rejected her.

But Elizabeth had learnt to think out of the box and she found a devious way out: becoming an apothecary. At the time, the Society of Apothecaries did not bar women from taking their exams, so she did just that. In those days, apothecaries were allowed to be practising physicians, although it was less prestigious than an MD.

Elizabeth obtained her licence to practice medicine and saw her name enrolled in the Medical Register one year later; the first woman qualified in Britain to do so. But as soon as Elizabeth was granted her diploma, the Society of Apothecaries immediately changed their rules to require graduation from an accredited medical school—all of which excluded women—as a prerequisite for the apothecary degree. As a result, no other woman's name would be added to the Medical Register for the next twelve years, after which the rules were changed.

With the support of her father, Elizabeth opened a dispensary for women and children in London. Initially, nobody came. But when an outbreak of cholera broke out and male doctors were flooded with patients, those turned away began to come to her. In that first year, she treated 3,000 patients.

Elizabeth would not be content with an apothecary degree though. In another great display of determination, she taught herself French, since she had heard that French universities were more open to admitting women students; and so it was. In 1870, she graduated from the University of Sorbonne with a medical degree, being granted France's first ever medical degree for a woman.

She also got married. James Anderson, a businessman, was supportive of her career, and they enjoyed what by all accounts was a long and happy marriage. They had three children, two of whom survived. Elizabeth would go on to be a strong advocate of a woman's right to both work and have a family.

By 1872, Elizabeth was back in the UK. The public had begun to thaw towards women doctors, swayed by Blackwell's visits and a clutch of other women medical students. Elizabeth's dispensary was renamed

the New Hospital for Women and Children, specialising in gynaecology, and to her great joy, her mentor Elizabeth Blackwell began to
teach there.

Then, in 1874, Elizabeth, along with Blackwell, Sophia Jex-Blake
and other women physicians, set up the London School of Medicine
for Women (LSM). It was the only teaching hospital at the time to
train women. The LSM would go on to train many Indian women to
be doctors, including Rukhmabai Raut.

At the inauguration of the LSM, Elizabeth Garrett Anderson made
a singular speech, an interesting illustration of her radical thoughts.
Unlike many women doctors, she did not believe that women automatically were the best choice to treat other women. In her speech, she
said, 'It is often said, for instance, that women will understand women's
ailments so much better than men do. I fancy this is only true in a very
partial and limited sense, and that it is most undesirable that medical
women themselves should place much confidence in it. No one would
say, for instance, that a horse or a dog would make a better veteri-
nary doctor than a man.' Instead, she argued, women doctors would
understand a disease because of their knowledge and intelligence, not
because of any 'occult sympathy' with the subject.[23]

She also had unorthodox views on the subject of female doctors
balancing family and work. As a working mother, she thought that female
doctors might not be able to take on as much work as men because they
had more family responsibilities, but also thought this was unimportant.
'Quality, not quantity' would make them popular, she argued.[24]

In 1876 came the triumph she and other women doctors had
waited so patiently for: The UK Medical Act finally allowed—though
not compelled—universities to admit women. The great fight was over.

Elizabeth Garrett Anderson died on 17 December 1917. She
could look back on a life of quiet yet awe-inspiring achievement. In
her no-nonsense manner, she had helped a generation of women in the
Empire to become doctors.

The Edinburgh Seven:
The Women Denied Degrees After Years Of Study

In April 2019, the University of Edinburgh corrected a terrible injustice of 150 years: it finally gave its first female students their degrees.

In 1869, seven women became the first female medical students enrolled at any British university, when they began studying at the University of Edinburgh. These seven were Sophia Jex-Blake, Edith Pechey, Isabel Thorne, Matilda Chaplin, Helen Evans, Emily Bovell and Mary Anderson—collectively known as the Edinburgh Seven. These women were callously denied their degrees, despite studying for three years and passing their examinations with honours.

Today, a plaque in the university with their names acknowledges the ill treatment of the Seven, and commemorates their courage in overcoming bigotry and discrimination. The tale of the Edinburgh Seven was a classic instance of how women medical students continued to meet resistance from envious male students, even after the examples set by the two Elizabeths: Blackwell and Garrett Anderson.

The Seven first came together after Sophia Jex-Blake put an ad in *The Scotsman*. Jex-Blake was a fiery, determined woman, who would later earn the label 'difficult' and take pride in it. She was born in 1840, at the beginning of the Victorian age, in a loving but conservative family. Early Victorian women were expected to stay at home, make good marriages and rear children. But Jex-Blake was a rebel.

Her childhood school reports and letters by her parents describe her consistently as 'wilful', 'tempestuous' and 'spirited'—code for girls who would not do as they were told. Her school friends too were intimidated by her confidence. 'Sophy is certainly excessively clever, but unfortunately knows it, and makes a point of showing it off on every possible occasion,' wrote one friend of her. 'Rather too fond of her own opinion,' wrote another, snidely.[25]

Her parents struggled to handle a girl who was clearly way ahead of her time. She convinced her parents to let her study at Queens

College. After only two months, the brilliant Jex-Blake was asked to work part-time as a maths tutor at the college, a great honour, but her father would not allow her to accept pay. Victorian women, even brilliant ones, did not work for money; they were supported by their menfolk.

The loving yet reproachful letters written by her father indicate Jex-Blake's struggle to win over her protective parent in particular and society in general. 'Dearest,' wrote her father. 'Take the post as one of honour and usefulness, and I shall be quite glad. But to be paid for the work would alter the thing completely, and lower you in the eyes of almost everybody.' Sophia's response was heartfelt and moving in its passion. 'I believe I am particularly well suited to teaching,' she wrote, adding that it was 'right and natural' that she take the payment, which was 5 shillings an hour. 'Why should I not take it? You as a man did your work and received your payment, and no one thought it any degradation. Why should the difference of my sex alter the laws of right and honour?' Sophia also mentioned the 'honest and particularly justifiable pride' of earning and asked why she should be deprived of it. Her father's response was to offer to send her the money she would have got by tutoring, and to promise her a good fortune if she were to be married the day after.[26]

Sophia declined the offer of money from her father, but after a series of letters, she clearly tired of the battle, and agreed to not take any teaching fees, for that term at any rate, though she reserved her right to be paid in the future.

The next few years were a time of confusion for Sophia. She was brilliant and driven, and initially she wanted to be a teacher, certainly a more acceptable profession for women of the time. To that end, she travelled to Boston to learn more about women's education. There, meeting the still tiny but growing number of women doctors, the ambitious idea of entering the medical profession began to take hold. She applied to Harvard Medical School, but they rejected her. Over the next three years, she kept trying, but they were firm. Sophia met the Blackwell sisters, who promised to help her, but before anything could happen to that end, her father died. A disconsolate Sophia decided to return to the UK.

Once back, she applied to the University of Edinburgh. There were four bodies that needed to approve her application. Three agreed, but the fourth rejected her on the flimsy grounds that it was too difficult to carry out 'temporary arrangements in the interests of one lady'. She was deeply disappointed. She kept a stiff upper lip in public, but in private, she wrote to her friend, 'It is very unusual and seems very hard... to repeat endless arguments to an endless succession of people that took so very much out of one.'[27] But she had her sympathisers, many of them male professors at the college.

Soon, an even more powerful advocate for Sophia came forward: *The Scotsman* newspaper. *The Scotsman* was a very influential paper, but also not known for its support of the weaker sections of society. It was conservative and insular, often supporting Scottish values, which were old-fashioned in those days. As the Scottish doctor and writer Margaret Todd wryly put it, when talking about the paper's self-absorption, 'It used to be said in those days, that when the North Pole was discovered, a Scotsman would be found sitting on it, and it might have been added that the Scotsman would prove to be engrossed in the newspaper that bore his name.' When *The Scotsman* decided to write about her campaign in its pages, it was a true game changer for Sophia. Meanwhile, her sympathisers urged her to put out an advertisement in the paper asking more women to join her in applying to the university. She did exactly that.

Six women came forward: Isabel Thorne, Edith Pechey, Mary Anderson, Emily Bovell, Matilda Chaplain and Helen Evans. Most of the women were disarmingly modest and self-deprecating, as they had been taught to be. Wrote Edith to Sophia, 'Do you think anything more is requisite to ensure success than moderate abilities and a good share of perseverance? I believe I may lay claim to these, together with a real love of the subjects of study, but as regards any thorough knowledge of these subjects at present, I fear I am deficient in most.'[28] The diffident Edith would go on to top the college in chemistry, and years later, would become the chief medical officer at the Madame Cama Hospital in Mumbai, where she would mentor a generation of Indian women.

In October 1869, the women sat the matriculation exam, for which they had to pass English, Latin, mathematics and other subjects. The examination was in two parts. Of the 152 candidates who sat the exam on 19 October 1869, five were women. Four of the women placed within the top seven. By November 1869, the University of Edinburgh became the first British university to admit women.

The women had to have separate classes from the men and pay higher tuition because these classes were smaller, but they studied the same subjects and followed the same rules. With classic understatement, but also bubbling over with joy, Sophia wrote in a letter to her friend, 'It is a grand thing to enter the very first British university opened to women, isn't it?'[29]

But the triumph was short-lived. In March 1870, the brilliant Edith Pechey won the Hope scholarship for standing in the top four in chemistry and physics. Her achievement made male teachers resentful and angry. Leading the campaign against the women was the powerful Robert Christison, who was staunchly against women in medicine. Christison thought that male students would be discouraged if they had to compete with brilliant women. Other teachers were affected by his views and Edith was denied the scholarship on the flimsy grounds that she had not attended the chemistry class taught to the men.

There was a mass outcry and considerable sympathy for Edith in the popular press, and there arose a debate as to whether the women should be allowed in mixed classes. However, Christison and his supporters continued to argue that women were fit by nature only to be midwives. Resentment built against the seven women. By the summer of 1870, the male students were howling and jeering at the women, shutting doors in their faces. The normally phlegmatic Edith wrote of how she was called 'a whore' in the street.[30] Later, many medical women in several other countries would be called by this epithet, the easiest way to try and put a woman in her place.

In November 1870, things came to a head, in what came to be called The Surgeons' Hall Riot. Sophia wrote about the events: 'As soon as we came in sight of the (University) gates, we found a dense mob filling up the roadway in front of them, comprising some dozen of the lowest class of our fellow students, many more of the same class from the University, a certain number of street rowdies, and some hundreds of gaping spectators… The gates were slammed in our faces by a number of young men, who stood within smoking and passing about bottles of whisky, while they abused us in the foulest possible language…'[31]

A gallant fellow student pulled the door open, and the women entered quickly, where they went to the anatomical classroom for an exam. Suddenly, a helpless sheep was pushed inside by the rioters. 'Let it remain,' said a doctor who supported the women. 'It has more sense than those who sent it there.' On their way out, and over the next few days, the women were protected by a stalwart bodyguard of male students, armed with sticks.

However, regardless of the support of these few men, there was a movement to deny the women their degrees.

Sophia's bell pull was wrenched off five times and a firecracker fixed to her door. 'The filthiest possible anonymous letters were sent to several of us; and the climax was when students took to waylaying us and shouting indecencies after us, making use of anatomical terms which they knew we could not fail to understand, while the police were equally certain not to do so.'[32]

Meanwhile, the women students were excluded from several

areas of the university, including the infirmary. An article in *The Edinburgh University Magazine* of February 1871, 'Female Education in Medicine', recommended that 'these female students offer their services as students, dressers, and clerks'. It concludes: 'Let us here, however, simply in self-defence state our firm belief that it is a sign not of advancing but of decaying civilisation when women force themselves into competition with the other sex.'[33]

By 1873, the women had lost. The Court of Session supported the university's right to refuse the women degrees, even though they had completed the course. Frankly, ruled the court, they should never have been admitted in the first place. The university was thus absolved of all responsibility. The women had wasted three years of their lives.

But Sophia, as always, had a plan B. She remained undaunted. In 1874, less than a year's time, she started the London School of Medicine for Women, along with Elizabeth Garrett Anderson, the formidable Blackwell sisters, Isabel Thorne and others of the Seven. The funds for the school were raised by thirteen contributors, most of them parents and well-wishers of the women, who contributed 100 pounds each. In 1874, 1,300 pounds was enough to rent a modest house and garden in Henrietta Street, a house that the tireless Sophia found by tramping the streets.

The London School of Medicine had fourteen students, and was the world's first medical school entirely for women. The fledgling school's first problem was that its degree was not recognised; the second that there was no qualifying examination open to its students. By 1876, when the first batch of women were nearing the completion of their degrees, the outlook was still 'gloomy'. As Isabel Thorne described it, the 'women seemed as far as ever from their goal'. But finally, in 1876, that which the Edinburgh Seven had battled so long and hard for finally happened: The UK Medical Act finally allowed all medical authorities to licence all qualified applicants, irrespective of gender. Shortly afterwards, the school entered into an agreement with the Royal Free Hospital to conduct clinical studies there. However, it took another sixteen years for the stubborn University of Edinburgh to admit women.

Five of the original seven—including Sophia—were granted MDs abroad in the late 1870s, either in Berne or Paris.

Women flocked to the London School of Medicine. Rukhmabai Raut was the first Indian woman to attend, and she was followed by many others, including the notable Jerusha Jhirad.

It seemed appropriate that when the University of Edinburgh finally awarded Sophia her degree in 2019, seventy-seven years after her death, it was accepted on her behalf by Nepali student Simran Piya. Piya said that before learning about the Seven, she took the ability to study medicine and get an education for granted. Learning about them helped her realise how female medical students got the opportunity to study.

The message of the Seven continues to resonate. Said Piya, 'I hope to take forward the legacy that the Edinburgh Seven established and continue to fight for their endeavours by being a positive female role model in a field like cardiology, and by volunteering in countries like Nepal where the gender divide in education is still a problematic issue in remote areas of the country.'[34]

CHAPTER TWO

The Good Wife

Anandibai Joshi

'If this life is so transitory like a rose in bloom, why should one depend upon another? Every one must not ride on another's shoulders, but walk on his own feet.'

A thirteen-year-old girl was being beaten by her thirty-year-old husband. This was not unusual for the India of 1878, when a husband's word was considered law. What was unusual, however, was the reason—she had been found cooking, not studying. As one biographer put it, 'The neighbourhood was agog: husbands beat wives for not cooking—but whoever had heard of a wife being beaten for cooking when she should have been reading?'[35]

This girl was Anandibai Joshi, who by twenty-one would become the first Indian woman to be a doctor. She would cross the dreaded kaala paani—black water (here it means to cross the ocean, which was forbidden for higher castes, otherwise they would lose their caste)—to study at the Women's Medical College of Pennsylvania (now Drexel University) at a time when most Hindu women never left their homes. She would do this alone, leaving her controlling husband behind and risking excommunication from her caste. She would resist immense pressure to convert to Christianity, despite the fact that all higher education for women was spearheaded by Christian institutions. And to do all this, she would pay a heavy price.

Anandibai walked a perilous tightrope between patriarchy and emancipation, and often it was difficult to tell which was which. Her chameleon-like character would confound her observers and biographers. A number of Marathi biographies were written about her. The American feminist writer and reformer Caroline Wells Healey Dall would also write a detailed, if cringingly orientalist, biography in 1888. Some saw Anandibai as a puppet of her husband Gopalrao Joshi; others saw in her letters a canny and intelligent woman who forged her own path. The truth perhaps lay somewhere in between.

'Joy Of My Heart'

Anandibai was born on 31 March 1865, the fifth of nine children, to a Brahmin family in Kalyan, then part of Pune. Her birth name was Yamuna. Healey Dall described her, mortifyingly, as the 'little brown baby whose future no one suspected.'[36]

Anandibai did not have a happy childhood. Her mother Gangabai was an authoritarian, abusive woman. 'My mother never spoke to me affectionately. When she punished me, she was wont to use not just a small rope or thong, but always stones, sticks, and live charcoal. Truly she never understood the duties of a mother, nor did I experience the love which a child naturally feels for its mother. This memory hurts me a great deal,' wrote Anandibai.[37]

With such a terrible childhood, the child Yamuna would look expectantly to her husband for love, support and guidance, and it was not long before this materialised. Yamuna was married at the age of nine to a man of twenty-six, already a widower, and renamed Anandibai, or 'joy of my heart'. A vast difference in age between bride and groom was common at the time, and yoking the fortunes of a child to a fully grown man—with one wife behind him already—was considered perfectly acceptable.

The man who would come to dominate and shape her life was the unusual Gopal Vinayak Joshi. He was a clerk in the postal department, and a man who was passionate about women's education—later, some would say a step too passionate. As a man who had tried and failed to make something of himself, he would use Anandibai as a way to get fame and adulation.

That we know anything about Anandibai at all is thanks to the numerous letters she wrote to Gopalrao while in the US, a very unusual thing to do for a woman of her time. As the writer and historian Meera Kosambi points out, 'Letterwriting was not a part of an Indian's daily routine. Besides, in an age when women's education or even literacy was frowned upon, it was a near impossibility.' Her letters—most likely a mix of Marathi and English—were preserved by a contemporary of hers, the Marathi writer Kashibai Kanitkar, who was a huge supporter of women's education. Kanitkar vividly described, from her own experience, how women who dared to read or write were shamed. 'If a woman picks up a paper, our elders feel offended, as though she has done something very shameful. If she receives a letter from her relatives, all the family feels dishonoured. If a woman's name appears in a newspaper, if her essay is published, if she stammers out a few words at a women's gathering, she is certain to be slapped with the gigantic charge of having tarnished the family's honour!'[38]

While women across India were treated like chattel, change was underway. A sweeping reform movement had begun. Initially, it was inspired by the spread of Western education in India, but soon Indian reformers began to analyse and question their own traditions. The reform movement was particularly strong in Maharashtra. Liberals such as M.G. Ranade, R.G. Bhandarkar and G.G. Agarkar spoke out in favour of widow remarriage and education for women. As early as 1848, the anti-caste couple Jotirao and Savitribai Phule set up a school in Pune for girls from all castes, despite huge opposition and abuse from conservative Brahmins.

Influenced by Western marriages, many reformers wanted their wives to be educated, giving rise to many progressive Maharashtrian couples. Often, even when the wife was reluctant, the husband would coax her into getting an education. When the reformer M.G. Ranade's first wife died, he wanted to marry a widow, but was forced by his family to marry the eleven-year-old Ramabai. Ranade then proceeded to educate his child bride—just as Jotirao Phule had educated Savitribai—and Ramabai grew into a formidable educationist in her own right. Together, they would set up the Huzurpaga Girls High School, which still survives today.

It is likely that Gopalrao was influenced by these reformist couples. It certainly explains his obsession with educating Anandibai. But educating your wife was a double-edged sword. Many a reformer was taken aback when his wife would unexpectedly become successful in her own right. Reform, as author and translator Aban Mukherji points out, was a male-dominated project, and the women had very little say in it. 'Many of the reformers were deeply ambivalent about the outcome of the reforms they themselves advocated. Such deep-rooted insecurity and anxiety led many reformers, such as Anandibai's husband, Gopalrao Joshi, to backtrack from or vacillate between the orthodox and reformist camps, propagating the education of women and widow remarriage one moment and then extolling child marriage (the next).'[39]

Trying to blend the best of East and West would be difficult for both Gopalrao and Anandibai. Gopalrao was also abusive. He would often beat the child Anandibai so severely that she would be covered with bruises. Later, Anandibai would write to him a heartbreaking letter that sharply revealed how difficult it was to balance Hindu custom and her own desire for emancipation.

> It is very difficult to decide whether your treatment of me was good or bad. If you ask me, I would answer that it was both. It seems to have been right in view of its ultimate goal; but, in all fairness, one is compelled to admit that it was wrong, considering its possible effects on a child's

mind. Hitting me with broken pieces of wood at the tender age of ten, flinging chairs and books at me and threatening to leave me when I was twelve, and inflicting other strange punishments on me when I was fourteen—all these were too severe for the age, body, and mind at each respective stage.

Anandibai went on to dispassionately lay out her limited options as a Hindu wife.

> If I had left you at that immature age, as you kept suggest-ing, what would have happened? I would have been lost. (And a number of girls have left their homes because of harassment from mothers-in law and husbands.) I did not do so because I was afraid that my ill-considered behaviour would tarnish my father's honour… And I requested you not to spare me, but to kill me. In our society, for centuries there has been no legal restraint between husbands and wives; and if it exists, it works against women! Such being the case, I had no recourse but to allow you to hit me with chairs and bear it with equanimity.
>
> A Hindu woman has no right to utter a word or to advise her husband. On the contrary, she has a right to allow her husband to do what he wishes and to keep quiet. Every Hindu husband can, with advantage, learn patience from his wife. I do understand that without you I would never have become what I am now, and I am eternally grateful to you; but you cannot deny that I was always calm.[40]

In 1878, when she was barely thirteen, a son was born to her, but he survived only ten days because of poor medical care and perhaps, her tender age. Many credit this incident for Anandibai's steely determination to learn medicine. Certainly, from then onwards her health was poor and she was constantly ill. Perhaps Gopalrao took it in his stride, but the death left a deep scar on his child bride. 'A child's death does no harm to its father,' she is reported to have said, 'but its mother does not want it to die.'[41]

The Carrot And The Stick

By 1878, news of the first women graduates in Britain had begun to trickle to India. Gopalrao, influenced by these, decided to educate Anandibai. At that point, there was no talk of her becoming a doctor; it would be daunting enough for her to simply get a primary education.

His methods of education were strictly carrot and stick, with more of the stick. So obsessed was Gopalrao with Anandibai's education that he would beat her if she attempted housework instead. Often, she would be deprived of food if she did not complete her reading for the day.

Gopalrao's radical views caused consternation in the community, and in both families. At the time, husband and wife were not supposed to spend time together and they were discouraged from even talking during the day, with the husband being out at work, the wife at home with her mother-in-law. But Gopalrao, while definitely the boss of the house, also wanted a companion. He would take Anandibai for long walks in Alibaug, causing a scandal in the neighbourhood. His own father protested. Gopalrao, ever the maverick, was unaffected.

Indeed, it was dangerous to go up against Gopalrao's sharp and unpredictable tongue. Anandibai's father Ganpatrao warned Gopalrao that educating a woman would only lead to her writing letters to outsiders, and even eloping with men. Women needed to be guarded at all costs, he said. Gopalrao replied tartly that such an event would relieve him of the burden of having to support a wife, at any rate.[42]

Anandibai attended a missionary school in Bombay because they were the only ones who encouraged the education of women at the time. She was reluctant to read the Bible, but Gopalrao convinced her that it was the only way to get an education. Gopalrao disliked the missionaries, but he was a realist, and thus not above ingratiating himself with them to get more opportunities.

Even in Bombay, supposedly the liberal capital of the country, Anandibai was harassed for being a Hindu girl who dared to go to school. She would later describe people laughing at her and jeering, and some going even further—'Others, sitting respectably in their verandas, made ridiculous remarks, and did not feel ashamed to throw pebbles at me. The shop-keepers and vendors spat at me, and made gestures too indecent to describe.'[43]

But these ordeals would make Anandibai tougher than most Brahmin women her age. She would become fluent in English, become independent and learn to do things in a way that women of the time could only dream of. Gopalrao would frequently let her travel alone to her family home, unheard of at a time when women were escorted everywhere by men.

Soon after, the news of British and Anglo-Indian women becoming doctors reached Gopalrao and he made up his mind that Anandibai would become one too. He realised that the only way to get help for Anandibai's education was to approach missionaries, much as he disliked them. In 1878, he wrote to Dr Royal Wilder, a well-known American missionary, expressing his willingness to move to America and work for Anandibai's education, and asking for support. 'Nothing is so important as female education for our elevation, morally and spiritually,' wrote Gopalrao, fervently. The letter was published in *The Missionary Review* and stirred up much debate about whether Indian women should be educated. Wilder offered to help, but only if the Joshis converted to Christianity.

This they flatly refused to do. It was a step too far for even the resourceful and relatively liberal Joshis.

At the time, most missionaries only wanted to educate Hindus who converted to Christianity. Caroline Wells Healey Dall wrote dryly, 'From a somewhat wide experience of male Hindus, I cannot consider their visits to the West profitable to themselves or others.'[44] Dall was not alone in her view. It was the rare Hindu who travelled overseas without converting, because Hinduism was looked upon as an inferior religion. Dall went on to sneer, 'It is not learning, intellect, subtlety or imagination that is wanting in the average Hindu; it is purity, faith and honesty.'

In later years, Gopalrao would enrage Dall and others by his constant criticism of missionaries and Christianity. But all that was yet to come. The Joshis had to put their plans on hold, but then they had an unbelievable, almost unimaginable, stroke of luck. Two years later, the old issue of *The Missionary Review* was lying in a dentist's office in New Jersey, where it was picked up by Mrs Theodicia Carpenter, another missionary but a less rigid one. Carpenter was moved by the brutal rejection of Gopalrao because of his religion. Early in March 1880, a full two years after Gopalrao had written to Wilder, Carpenter wrote to Gopalrao, a small, random act of kindness, which changed all their lives forever.

'My Dear Aunt': Anandibai Finds A Friend

Anandibai and Mrs Carpenter began an unlikely and loving correspondence, each trying to teach the other their cultures, with Anandibai calling Mrs Carpenter, 'My dear aunt'. In Mrs Carpenter, Anandibai found the loving, kind, maternal figure she had never had.

Anandibai would write about Hindu manners, customs and rites. She would send pictures, magazines and even flowers and seeds to her new friend. Her courtly, slightly old-fashioned English greatly impressed Mrs Carpenter. In one instance, Anandibai sent out a gift of til seeds, for 'making comfits', and then these were followed by parcels of buckwheat, millets, peas and beans.

They would engage in spirited discussions over whose culture was better. In these fascinating letters, Anandibai chafed against patriarchal Hindu customs, but also resented what she saw as the arrogance and condescension of missionaries, who presumed they knew Hindu women best.

Around this time, Gopalrao decided to seek a transfer to Calcutta, because he had heard that the postal department there was offering jobs to women. But when they arrived there, they found it even more conservative than Pune, with the purdah system (a religious and social practice of female seclusion common among some Muslim and Hindu communities) playing a huge role in this perception. People would stare and jeer at the couple. Frustrated, Anandibai wrote to Mrs Carpenter, 'There is so much of the zenana system (a Muslim social institution in which separate spaces are assigned to women, who are kept in seclusion) that a woman can scarcely stand in the presence of her relatives, much less before her husband. Her face is always veiled. She is not allowed to speak to any man, much less to laugh with him.'[45]

Anandibai had begun to read widely and analyse her readings in a manner rare for women of that time. She wrote of how she was compelled to read the Bible in school by a missionary. 'As a whole I have nothing to say against the Bible except the assertion "He that shall believeth shall be saved and he who believeth shall not be damned." I have all along found the missionaries very headstrong and contemptuous of the faiths of others. How arbitrary would it be if I were to say that all you believed was nonsense and all I believed was just and proper?'

In the same letter, Anandibai displayed a remarkable and liberal sentiment for the time. 'My dear friend, I have nothing to despise. The whole universe is a lesson to me. I am required by duty to respect every creed and sect and value its religion. I therefore read the Bible with as much interest as I read my own religious books.'[46]

Anandibai's growing awareness of the deep unfairness of Hindu customs—especially rigid Brahminism—and her longing for more freedom is apparent. In one of her earliest letters to Carpenter, she wrote, 'We women have the same dress for all the seasons. We never put on warm clothes as it is considered indecent, nor do we wear shoes or boots as we seldom go outdoors. In short, all these luxuries are for men, who feel cold, warm and autumn [weather] and not for women who are supposed to be impervious to all these changes of climate. Should we not envy you then?' In another letter, she wrote resentfully of how women in India 'have no letters to write, or books to read. They do not receive or make calls, except among their own female relatives.'[47] It seems apparent that Anandibai yearned for a life free of these restraints, one where she might read, study and savour the freedoms that American women enjoyed.

Standing On Her Own Feet

After two years of exchanging letters, Mrs Carpenter suggested that Anandibai come to America. Anandibai responded eagerly. No longer was she so reliant on Gopalrao. She said that she was quite willing to go alone to America, because her husband had an old mother and brothers to care for. Besides, they could not afford for both of them to go. 'Considering the future prospects of my life as a physician I must make up my mind to be separated from my husband.' Her letter went on to say things which were remarkably revolutionary for a secluded upper-caste Hindu woman. 'If this life is so transitory like a rose in bloom, why should one depend upon another? Every one [sic] must not ride on another's shoulders, but walk on his own feet.'[48]

Over the next few months, Anandibai faced considerable opposition to her decision from both Indians and foreigners. So loud was the outcry against her that Gopalrao decided to publicly state their plans in the College Hall at Serampore, hoping to quell the opposition of the community. But at the last minute, Anandibai decided to make the statement herself, defying the custom that Brahmin women were not to appear in public. It is impossible to overstate the significance of her appearance before a crowd of men at a time when Indian women never left the house. It was courage of a rare and incredible kind.

On 24 February 1883, she addressed a motley group of Indians and Europeans. Her speech was later turned into a little pamphlet. Anandibai gave her speech in English, on the subject of 'My future visit to America and public inquiries regarding it'. She addressed a number of questions she had been asked. 'Why do I go to America?' she said. 'Are there no means to study in India? Why do I go alone? Why should I do what is not done by any of my sex?'

'I go to America because I wish to study medicine. There are some female doctors in India from Europe and America, who, being foreigners, have not been of such use to our women as they might. It is very natural that Hindu ladies who love their own country and people should not feel at home with the natives of other countries.'[49] Anandibai went on to explain that the restricted freedoms allowed to non-Christian, non-Brahmo women in India, the social strictures against her and the harassment she had faced, made it near impossible for her to study in India.

'Shall I not be excommunicated when I return to India? I do not fear it in the least.' Bravely, she continued, 'Why should I be cast out when I have determined to live there exactly as I do here? I propose to myself to make no change in my customs and manner, food and dress. I will go as a Hindu and come back here to live as a Hindu.'[50] This she was to do, wearing a sari and being vegetarian until the end of her stay, to the dismay of many Western missionaries who had hoped she would convert.

Talking about the dangers of the journey, Anandibai said, 'Some say that those who stay at home are happy, but where does their happiness lie? In going to foreign countries, we may enlarge our comprehension, perfect our knowledge.' Then she concluded with her reasons to want study medicine. 'You ask me, why I should do what is not done by any of my sex? To this I can only say that society has a right to our work as individuals. If anything seems best for all mankind, each one of us should try to bring it about.'[51]

This powerful speech moved many, and prompted donations from well-wishers. Selling her bangles to fund her journey, like so many Indian women would do before and after her for money, Anandibai finally sailed on 7 April 1883, on the ship *City of Calcutta*, with a number of missionaries. The journey was gruelling and difficult, especially because she was determined to stick to her vegetarian diet. She lived in a state of near starvation, 'rejecting the dried fishes, long-long bones, soup, and things composed of old vegetables, stalks and half-rotten potatoes'.[52]

It would be sixty days before she arrived in New York, where she was met by Mr and Mrs Carpenter, who had travelled from Roselle, New Jersey, to meet their adopted daughter.

Land Of The Free And Home Of The Brave

Anandibai's first days in New York were a blur of activity, as she was shown off to curious American women. 'A visit to Tiffany's gave her great pleasure.'[53]

Then came a massive feast for her friends in New Jersey. The floor was decorated with 'powders brought from India', which one must assume were rangolis. The ladies were dressed in saris from Anandibai's wardrobe. The strictly vegetarian feast had eighteen dishes of, as the superior Dall described, 'peculiar Hindu cookery'. To the bewilderment of the guests, there was no cutlery at all. 'Anandibai would pick up a morsel, bring it a few inches from her plate, and then with a few dexterous twists of her fingers toss into her mouth. To miss, she said, would be vulgar,'[54] wrote Healey Dall. Sadly, no photographs survive of this riotous meal.

Her first few months were terribly lonely. Not surprisingly, given how large a part Gopalrao played in her life, she missed him. Much of

her time was spent writing letters. In August 1883, she wrote a poignant letter to him.

'I cannot describe the joy I feel on receiving your news so frequently.
It is the only avenue for contact with you, for which I shall always be
grateful to God... Day and night, I think of writing to you, and you
never leave my heart!'[55]

Then came Anandibai's admission into the Women's Medical
College (WMC) of Pennsylvania. In her application letter to the then
dean, Dr Rachel Bodley, Anandibai cleverly emphasised the lack of
medical aid for Indian women, saying that she needed to help those
who could not help themselves. 'The determination which has brought
me to your country against the combined opposition of my friends
and caste ought to go a long way towards helping me to carry out
the purpose for which I came, that is to render to my poor suffering
country women the true medical aid they so sadly stand in need of and
which they would rather die than accept at the hands of a male physician. My soul is moved to help the many who cannot help themselves,'
she wrote.[56]

She added that she had 70 dollars with her, and her husband
would send her 20 dollars per month; and that she had learnt to read
and speak in seven Indian languages, had been once through English
grammar and had studied as far as division in mathematics.[57]

Dr Bodley, who had become dean of the college in 1874, was an
unusual woman, every bit as unusual as the girl she had responded
to. She was a professor of chemistry, and in 1862 had catalogued an
extensive plant collection at the Cincinnati Female Seminary, a feat
that won her many admirers. She was also deeply religious, an evangelical Christian from a Quaker family, and a supporter of medical
missionaries.

No doubt, Bodley would have preferred a Christian candidate,
or one less determined to cling to her roots. Still, she was impressed
by Anandibai and championed her, despite the fact that she was a

'Hindoo'. Eventually, the WMC decided to admit her. Dr Bodley held a grand reception for her with over five hundred people that Anandibai would excitedly detail to Gopalrao, writing about how she wore her 'red Pitamber sari'.[58]

The Women's Medical College Of Pennsylvania

What would Anandibai have seen when she entered the graciously proportioned WMC building? A group of mostly white women, but yet more diverse than in any other medical college of the time. In 1885, more than twenty women from Asia, Latin America and the Middle East attended WMC, a number which would rise in later years. Some of the women she met were as alien a sight as she was, and equally conservatively dressed in long shirtwaist dresses, 'leg of mutton' sleeves and hair elaborately piled up in chignons. There were few safety measures: no goggles, helmets or gloves.[59]

Fittingly for Anandibai, the WMC was a pioneer of its time too. WMC was founded in 1850—a year after Elizabeth Blackwell became America's first woman doctor—exclusively to train women to become doctors. It was founded by a group of liberal Quakers, the same sect that had encouraged Blackwell, and that had a history of supporting women's education.

At the time, the idea of women in medicine was roundly ridiculed, sometimes even by other women. 'I shall not submit my pulse to anything that wears a bonnet,' concluded a letter to *The Boston Journal* in 1850. It was written by a woman, the popular women's columnist and humourist, Fanny Fern. 'We consider the needle a much more appropriate weapon in the hands of woman than the scalpel,'[60] she continued. Fern may have intended humour, but there is no doubt that a strong prejudice against women being doctors existed.

At its inauguration, one of the founders, Dr Joseph Longshore, gave a fiery speech, emphasising that the denial of medical education to women was profoundly unjust. 'That the exercise of the healing art, should be monopolized solely by the male practitioner... can neither be sanctioned by humanity, justified by reason, [nor] approved by ordinary intelligence; prejudice, bigotry, and selfishness may dispute woman's claim to the high calling, but an enlightened liberty, and intelligent sense of justice, never.'[61]

The first two deans were Quaker men, but from 1866, women acted as deans for the college. Bodley was tireless in her efforts to get positive publicity for the women graduates: 'big them up', as it were. In 1881, two years before Anandibai entered the WMC, Bodley presented 'The College Story', the results of a survey into the post-graduation lives of the 244 living alumni of the Women's Medical College. The survey found that, of the 189 women who responded, 88 per cent were still practising medicine, with only eight women citing 'domestic duties' as their reason for leaving the medical practice.[62] This was a fitting response to opponents of female medical education, who claimed that women would simply give up the practice once they married.[63]

Nevertheless, even twenty years after the college was founded, there was still prejudice against women doctors. In November 1869, there was a turning point for women students, an incident which went down in history as 'The Jeering'. A group of about thirty-four women students from WMC were harassed, hissed at, called names and spat at by male medical students when they attended a clinical lecture at Pennsylvania Hospital. The men would not allow the teacher to speak; instead they howled, shouted and catcalled the women to get them to move out of the hall. The women sat on, unperturbed and resolute, covered in tobacco juice. The incident was condemned as an 'outrage' and 'disgraceful' by local papers, some of whom suggested that women and men should be taught in separate classes.[64]

But later that same month, a piece appeared in *The New Republic*, purporting to show the 'other side'. The author claimed that the women had never been booed, jeered or insulted, but then rather undermined his own argument by getting exceptionally angry, calling the thirty-four women 'a shameless herd of sexless beings who dishonour the garb of ladies' and a 'bearded set of non-blushers who infest the rights of regular students.'[65]

All this controversy only made the women more resolute. Later, one of the determined students, Sarah Hibbard, wrote, 'But if these poor fellows had sought to do us a lifelong favour, they could not have done it more effectively than in their conduct towards us during those sessions.'[66]

The first black woman medical student, Sarah Mapps Douglas, would enrol at the WMC just two years later, though she would not graduate. In 1867, the college would go on to produce Rebecca Cole, only the second black woman to get an MD in the country. The country's first Native American woman to become a doctor, Susan La Flesche Picotte, graduated from WMC in 1889. Like most of their graduates, she returned home to her people, and practised for years on the reservation.

By 1904, the college would have women graduates from across the world, including India, China, Jamaica, Switzerland, Brazil and Russia. This was an era when women were still considered unfit for medicine because they were easily hysterical and weak. Indeed, at the time, women could not even vote. So, to get access to education was ground-breaking.

Why did so many foreign women attend the WMC? One reason may have been that American medical colleges at the time were fairly easy to get into. Only in the 1920s did American medical colleges finally begin to require a college degree. This, of course, was why Anandibai could enter with only a rudimentary education, while her successors would need college degrees in the sciences.

Another reason was the presence of US missionaries in many countries. Most of the women at WMC were sponsored by churches, and would return to their countries to work for missionary organisations.

Anandibai would be the brave exception, though even she had reached Pennsylvania with the help of missionaries like Mrs Carpenter.[67]

The foreign women at WMC were much feted and Dr Bodley was smart enough to know that they would help bring publicity for the college. She organised a series of receptions, gatherings and speeches. One of the most famous photographs of Anandibai is one from the dean's reception of 1885, with Keiko Okami, the second woman doctor from Japan, and Sabat Islambooly, the first woman doctor from Syria. Later, Okami would return to Japan, where she would head a department of gynaecology, only to resign when the then Japanese emperor refused to meet her because of her gender. She would go on to practise independently for twenty years. Nothing is known of Islambooly's career after leaving the WMC. In the photograph, all three are dressed in their magnificent national dresses. Okami, in an elaborate kimono, gazes to her right. Islambooly, weighed down with heavy Syrian jewellery, looks thoughtful. Anandibai, dressed in a sari, gazes impassively into the camera. Her expression is solemn and unreadable.[68]

By this time, Anandibai had become an emblem of pride in India, even amongst Hindu conservatives. Her steely resolve to not convert to Christianity, while surrounded by missionaries, was much admired. Her determination to cling to the traditions of Hindu womanhood—vegetarianism, conservative dress, wifely devotion—was similarly praised in *Kesari* and other conservative journals. Later, another woman who tried to follow in her footsteps would be savagely reviled by these same conservatives. But for now, Anandibai became an unlikely symbol of Mahratta pride. Bal Gangadhar Tilak wrote to her offering her 100 rupees, and calling her one of the greatest women of the modern era.[69]

We have very little information on her studies, but it is clear they were exacting. Her first year subjects were chemistry, physiology, anatomy, materia medica, surgery and histology. During the second year, these subjects would be continued and four more added.

Nevertheless, Anandibai would spend a great deal of time writing letters, as much as two hours a day. It was not unusual for her to receive seven letters a day, from Gopalrao, family members such as her brother-in-law and well-wishers.[70] On a typical day, she rested seven to eight hours, spent two hours on letter-writing, an hour and a half on meals, half an hour on visits, half an hour on her toilette, and the rest of the time on lectures and studies.[71]

While constantly ill, the delicate Anandibai was nevertheless tougher than she appeared. 'I met a mad woman for the first time in the College Hospital,' she wrote to Gopalrao. It was after a post-mortem dissection demonstration by a professor and a senior classwoman. After it concluded, she was standing alone by the dissection table, next to the corpse with its organs revealed, when she found herself confronted with a woman who Anandibai said, 'From her general demeanour, I had already guessed that she was quite insane. She seemed to be stronger than I, and capable of using the instruments lying there if she wanted to. I did not move from that spot, because I thought she would follow me, but I was not in the least afraid of her.' Her attendant came to take her away even as Anandibai was inching away from the scene, on the advice of a terrified Mrs Smith.[72]

The Juggling Act

Anandibai's new-found independence both gladdened and infuriated Gopalrao. The wife he had groomed since she was nine was now making her own decisions and was much admired by those who surrounded her. It left Gopalrao feeling powerless and deserted. Anandibai would become involved in a constant juggling act to placate him and yet retain her own identity.

An endless source of conflict was Anandibai's dress. She was the first foreigner in the WMC to keep her native dress; the other foreign women had long since adopted the American way of dress. But even this was not good enough for Gopalrao.

Anandibai's resolve to not change her way of dress was severely tested by the harsh Philadelphia winters. The traditional nine-yard Maharashtrian sari with its exposed legs offered little protection against the brutal winds. So, she wore her sari Gujarati style. This simple act enraged Gopalrao, who saw it as giving up her Marathi roots. Anandibai was forced to go on the defensive. 'The Maharashtrian dress will be comfortable only in the summer and I feel it would be improper to change my costume [according to season], besides looking like a performer in different guises. I have resolved to keep the same manner of dress all the time. As soon as I leave this country, I will dress in the Maharashtrian style; that is my firm decision,' she wrote.[73]

On another occasion, after seeing a photograph of her, Gopalrao wrote a furious letter, alleging that Anandibai had not covered her shoulders and bosom adequately. A resigned Anandibai wrote back, humouring him like a mother does her child, 'In your letter you have criticised the blouse I wore in the photograph, but I promise you I never thought of it. I am sorry it made you unhappy,' she wheedled. 'The *padar* (edge) of the *pitambar* fell off my shoulder not because of carelessness, but inadvertently. I was not aware of it, nor was anybody else. That is why the photograph was taken as it was. I know only too well that the fault will be mine, if I do anything to incur public censure. Usually I do not act without proper consideration. I think it better to cut off the organ which is likely to harm the whole body. I wear my current dress only for protecting my health.'[74]

In 1884, she fell ill of diphtheria, one of the first of many illnesses she continued to be plagued with. She eventually recovered, but her health remained fragile. That summer, Anandibai gave more evidence of the contradictions in her nature that exasperated feminists and pleased conservatives. She gave an address before the Ladies Missionary Society, backing the early marriage of women. Perhaps this was no surprise given Gopalrao's support for her education, and her complete dependence on him. Nevertheless, her new friends were shocked. Caroline Wells Healey Dall sought to defend her, 'All the happiness of her life had flowed from the instruction of her husband, and from the liberal sympathy which she supposed to move him in assisting her to come to this country.'[75]

The constant tension between East and West was evident in other areas too. In 1883, Anandibai wrote a fascinating list in her friend Mrs Carpenter's album, titled 'A Mental Photograph'. The list is very revealing of her character: an uneasy melange of Indian tradition and Western emancipation.

The initial entries are harmless and fun. For favourite poet, Anandibai listed Alexander Pope, Manu and Kalidasa, and for prose, Oliver Goldsmith, Thomas Macaulay and Shastree Chiploonkar. Her favourite character in history was, rather unusually, not an Indian but Richard Coeur de Lion. Yet her favourite book 'to take up for an hour' was the Bhagavad Gita. Her idea of misery, interestingly, was to 'follow one's own will', and yet her bête noire was 'slavery and dependence'. The answer to the question 'What is your most distinguishing characteristic?' was 'I have not yet found it'. That of her husband was 'benevolence', an odd choice of word for a man who beat her constantly. Her ideal pleasure was to be 'rewarded for what I do'.[76]

Meanwhile, Anandibai and Gopalrao argued about her future. Gopalrao wanted her to stay on in America, while he tried to join her, but Anandibai wanted to return to India. She reasoned that there was already a glut of women doctors in the US, who could not find work anyway because of discrimination. 'Many think it better not to have them. Men hate them.' Instead, Anandibai sketched ambitious plans to return to India, help the cause of women's health, set up a women's medical college and give lectures. 'Why leave a full plate to go begging elsewhere?' she argued.[77]

Anandibai's Battle Against Orientalism

As a Hindu woman in the US, Anandibai was constantly torn between the natural friendliness of Americans and her annoyance at their condescension, and often their orientalism. While Mrs Carpenter and Dr Rachel Bodley were kind to Anandibai, she met many American women who thought her stupid and downtrodden, as they did all Indian women.

When Anandibai was taken around on visits to intrigued Americans in neighbouring towns, they cosseted her like a doll. The gatherings were in equal parts enthralled and revolted by her religious symbols, her bindi, her nose ring, her dress and her customs.

Dall had her first—and what would prove to be her last—meeting with Anandibai in December 1884. The waspish Dall had a poor opinion of Hindus, but graciously allowed, 'In one respect from first to last, she was herself alone in the sweetest truthfulness, the most entire candour that ever belonged to a mortal, and I have good reason to think that is not a common Hindu trait.'[78]

Anandibai was diplomatic in person, but her letters reveal her frustration. In an exasperated letter to Gopalrao, she wrote about what she saw as the silly and patronising questions asked by many American women. 'One of the foolish questions asked by a woman doctor was, "Does India have many women?" She said, "I hear that it is your custom to kill a baby girl as soon as she is born! This country [America] has more women than men, but there must be relatively few women in India if female infants are killed." This is the wisdom and progress of the Westerners whom we praise so much! And so, if they imagine us to be the middle link between monkeys and humans, it would not be surprising! What a dreadful idea! I did not know that India is such a barbaric and cruel country!'[79]

Anandibai also found it immensely painful to be called a 'heathen'. She was compelled to defend her religious beliefs on many occasions.

'I feel no shame if they use the word in its literal sense. I would say that I too am an unbeliever. And I am proud of it...'

Seeing the relative freedom of American women prompted Anandibai to think carefully about the status of Indian women. As always, her pragmatism was at war with her innate nationalism. She wanted more freedom for Indian women—how could she not—but the superior airs of American women who knew nothing about her country or customs enraged her. 'We Indian women who are without status, deprived of our rights by men, and more backward in every way, are still better than them! It is worth remembering that being inherently weak, we have had to cultivate the typically Indian fortitude in order to protect morality, religion and intellect! Every nation should emulate Indian women and learn endurance from them. They may be superstitious, ignorant, misguided, or may hold wrong beliefs, but [they] can hardly be blamed. Since all laws, rules, customs, etc., are favourable to men, it is not surprising or improbable that the women have remained in this state.'[80]

Inwardly, Anandibai often ranted against the arrogance of American women, and the manner in which they believed their culture was always best. Her placid manner concealed a wicked sense of humour, often revealed only to her husband. In a letter to Gopalrao, she wrote, 'There is a new fashion of wearing girdles. Already the practice of tight-lacing makes it impossible to breathe freely, and now this fashion! This is the way to improve upon progress! If the Chinese bind their feet, it is because they are ignorant and idolaters. If Westerners do such things, it is because they are very advanced!'

Anandibai had hopes that Indian women might do better. 'I do not like to harp on the past; but unless the past and present are compared, the future cannot be predicted. We must also understand why, when and how men respected us or protected us from enemies, or deprived us of our rights. Instead of grieving about the present, or resenting the good fortune of others, one should concentrate on how to escape from ignorance.' She ended her long letter to Gopalrao with a sly dig at male privilege: 'Please note how often I have to beg your pardon so that you do not misunderstand me...'[81]

Perhaps as a frustrated reaction to these endless attacks on Indian culture, Anandibai's thesis was on 'Obstetrics amongst the Aryan Hindus'. The thesis explored and praised traditional Indian ways of pregnancy, childbirth and maternal health, citing Manu, Susruta and other such gurus. Some historians have seen the emphasis on the word 'Aryan' as evidence of Anandibai's increasing 'cultural nationalism', and as a defensive attempt to defend Indian medicine, which had been widely criticised. Her thesis was also careful to emphasise the positive aspects of Indian healthcare, leaving out any mention of the often dark and unhygienic rooms used for childbirth, the uneducated midwives and the superstitions which crowded out science.[82]

Anandibai Versus Ramabai: The Good Wife Versus The Rebel

It was at about this time that Anandibai met her polar opposite, Pandita Ramabai, a writer, activist and crusader for women's education. The two women were distantly related, 'cousins three times removed'. They left India at the same time, in the same month—Ramabai for the UK, Anandibai for the US. Yet, they never met until 6 March 1886, at the time of Anandibai's graduation.

The canny Dr Rachel Bodley realised that there could be no bigger publicity coup for the WMC than having two educated Hindu women unite in the US and talk about their journey. So, she wrote to Ramabai and invited her across the pond to attend the graduation. The two women were finally united in Bodley's living room.

The two women could not have been more different. Anandibai was a devout Hindu, supported child marriage and believed in her wifely duties. Ramabai was a savage critic of Hinduism, child marriage and the seclusion of Hindu women, and did not mince her words in saying, 'The complete submission of women under the Hindu law has converted them into slavery-loving creatures.' Anandibai had clung firmly to her religion. Ramabai had converted to Christianity soon after her arrival in London, in a move that shocked the orthodox Pune Brahmin community.

Ramabai was a rebel in every way. She had been born to a liberal father who had taken care to educate her well, in Sanskrit as well as in English. So vast was her Sanskrit learning that Calcutta University conferred the titles of 'Pandita' (an expert or scholar in any area of knowledge, but particularly Hindu scriptures and philosophy) and 'Saraswati'(the name of the Hindu goddess of knowledge) on her. She even married out of caste, but was widowed shortly afterwards, leaving her with a young daughter, Manorama.

Both women believed passionately in the education of their sex, but they went about it in very different ways: Ramabai, fierce, uncompromising, outspoken, and Anandibai, reticent, measured and careful not to give offence to the community. Ramabai had founded a society in Pune to build schools for girls, and then travelled widely to set up branches. She was a strong supporter of medical education for women. Indeed, she too had wanted to become a doctor, but was rejected in the UK because of her poor hearing. Instead, she became a professor of Sanskrit at that poshest and most British of institutions: the Cheltenham Ladies' College. Most importantly, she had achieved all this without the help of a man, extremely unusual for Hindu women of that time.

Not surprisingly, Ramabai had been warmly welcomed—even idolised—by Western missionaries. They gushed over her beauty, her chiselled features and large eyes, her learning, her genius for public speaking. 'Ramabai is strikingly beautiful,' enthused the unapologetically racist Caroline Wells Healey Dall. 'There is nothing else about her to suggest the Hindu.' So enthusiastic was Healey Dall that she felt the need to ask Anandibai about Ramabai's parentage.

'I cross-questioned Anandibai pretty closely about a possible mixture of blood. She acknowledged that there is a frequent crossing of the Mahratta blood by that of Cashmere.'[83]

While Anandibai was always looked upon with suspicion for her odd 'Hindoo' ways in the US, Ramabai was regarded with horror back home in India: for her conversion and her criticism of Hindu customs.

The Indian press sought to compare one with the other, too, especially after Ramabai's conversion, emphasising Anandibai's docile and religious temperament. An editorial in the Marathi weekly *Kesari* blatantly set one woman against the other: 'Mrs Anandibai Joshi's character is very different from Pandita Ramabai's. We strongly hope that this humble and well-behaved lady will acquire a good training in medicine as planned, and, without committing any lapse with regard to religion and conduct as the Sanskrit [Ramabai] did, return to this country and work for the welfare of her destitute country women in many ways. Those who have personally seen Mrs Anandibai recount that her temperament is not fickle, obstinate, or arrogant, but very submissive and deferential. Anandibai's letters give ample evidence of her faith in God, fear of sin, and love for her husband.'[84]

There was clearly intense pressure on Anandibai to convert. Most of her fellow students, including those from Asia, were converts to Christianity. Again and again, she was forced to defend herself, even to her own husband. Anandibai resolved to bend and not break, but was still frustrated that people continued to suspect her.

Anandibai too had been shocked by the news of Ramabai's conversion. In 1883, she wrote to Gopalrao, 'The account of Ramabai, if true, is very saddening. She has really brought a stigma to female education, religious faith, truth, etc. It is difficult to assess the extent to which it will obstruct female education.'[85] Later she wrote, exasperatedly, clearly weary of being compared to Ramabai, 'Ramabai is not Anandibai, and Anandibai is not Ramabai! The two are different individuals, created for different work. Even if I die, I will not act contrary to my beliefs. Ramabai is twenty times more learned than I.'[86] When the two women finally met, Anandibai was much impressed by Ramabai and her daughter Manorama. Despite the attempts to create a toxic rivalry between them, she tried to rise above it. Ramabai's speech at the WMC was attended by nearly six hundred people, and she went on to give more speeches across America, which unsurprisingly took her to its bosom.

Only a year later, Ramabai went on to write a brave and scandalous book, *The High Caste Hindu Woman*, which flayed Hinduism for its treatment of women: child marriages, ostracism of widows and the confinement of women to the home. The book became very popular in the US, because of its appeal to Americans to help Hindu women escape the zenana.

Ramabai would come to believe that the only way Indian women could be emancipated was to convert to Christianity. She returned to India in 1889 and set up a home for widows, Sharada Sadan. Initially secular, it would later become a controversial Christian organisation called Mukti Mission, which still exists today. The home would provide shelter for destitute girls and women, mostly widows and orphans. By 1900, there were 2,000 women living there. By 1908, the home had become an evangelical institution intended to train women to go out and propagate the word of the Bible.

Manorama would grow up to be every bit as passionate and unconventional as Ramabai. She too would join the cause of women's education. The two would die within a year of each other, having broken every rule in the book for Hindu women.

Gopalrao, The Eccentric

In 1885, towards the end of her course, Anandibai had to endure a much longed for and yet eventually difficult visitor: Gopalrao. For a while, Gopalrao, resentful of all the attention paid to his young wife, had been pondering about how to grab some of it for himself. He had been planning a trip for some time, but had been deterred by the cost. Eventually, the couple saved enough for the long journey.

Instantly, the lovely freedom and independence that Anandibai had enjoyed began to disappear, like air leaking slowly from a balloon. To put it mildly, the envious Gopalrao lost no opportunity to embarrass his wife. Anandibai had carefully, slowly, painstakingly built up a reputation as a sober, hard-working woman. In an instant, her eccentric husband came close to destroying it.

Gopalrao began his disastrous trip by giving a speech in San Francisco, where he criticised higher education for women, on the grounds that it made them unfit for the domestic duties of wives and mothers. When a person in the crowd shouted, 'I thought your own wife was studying medicine in Philadelphia', Gopalrao simply shrugged. 'Then he spread out his hands as if he would say, how could I help that?'[87] Later, when asked why he made the speech, he replied, 'Just for a little fun. I thought I would stir them up a little.'

Anandibai had to once again walk the fine line between her natural feelings of gratitude to her mentors and being a good Hindu wife. Gopalrao, probably chafing at having to accept charity from American missionaries, was loud in his opinions about Christianity and American culture. He thought it was degenerate, imperialist and saw no reason to keep his views to himself.

In June 1886, the *Index* paper reported on a debate on religion at which 'Gopalrao was introduced as "not... a member of the Brahmo Samaj, or of Reformed Hinduism, but... an adherent of the ancient Brahmanism". His address on "What is Lacking in Christianity" was liberally sprinkled with "substantiated" statements that Christianity lacked justice, righteousness, humanity, honesty of purpose and charity. It concluded: Though Christianity does not possess any noble attribute, yet this country is most prosperous and wealthy. As I said before, Christianity is the best fertilizer, but a most disgusting thing to look at.'[88]

Could he have said anything more embarrassing, given his wife had made it to America with the help of missionaries? 'Probably nothing in her life was so trying to Dr Joshi as the round of visits which now began in her husband's company. Alone I had known her more than once to interpose her gentle word, but before others her duty as a Hindu wife forbade her to speak,' wrote the keen observer Healey Dall, who watched as Anandibai became ever more self-effacing in Gopalrao's company.[89]

Gopalrao, meanwhile, got more and more confident and eager to express his opinions, even when nobody asked him. In March 1886, he wrote a letter to the *Index*, airing his views on Rukhmabai Raut's court case (whose life is discussed in detail in Chapter 4). At eleven, Rukhmabai had been married to a man much older than her; years later, she refused to move into his home, filed for divorce and was sentenced to a prison term. The case had caused immense outrage both in India and overseas. Gopalrao staunchly defended the simplicity and innocence of child marriages. 'We don't want your marriage system. We don't want your divorce. We don't want your swindles and frauds. Keep them all to yourselves. We don't envy you. But don't condemn our child marriage system and call us by hard names.'[90] Once more, the wide chasm between the Maharashtrian reformers' supposed ideals and the reality of their lives was exposed.

While Anandibai's friends and mentors were horrified by Gopalrao's rudeness, there was a certain bitter truth to his rants about evangelical Christianity and its role in aiding colonialism and imperialism. 'These greedy Christians did not go into the adjoining countries where there was nothing but sand and flint, but to those countries which abounded in gold and silver, and where industry was an honest pursuit and selfishness an unpardonable sin, and ingratitude a capital crime.' Gopalrao went further. 'I do not speak against Christ and his teachings, but I find his followers unworthy of the name. I have been with missionaries for the last twenty-two years. The more I look into their characters, the darker is the dye that stains them. Christians have manufactured all the vices, and exported them to countries where simplicity and innocence reigned.'[91]

However true some of Gopalrao's views may have been, they are likely to have caused deep agony to Anandibai, who had had no choice but to take help from missionaries to get where she was. Through it all, Anandibai remained silent and said nothing, either in writing or in person. Dr Bodley had this to say about Anandibai's dilemma, 'Ramabai's chapter on the married life of the Hindu woman reveals to the Western Reader what it was for this refined, intellectual person, whose faculties developed rapidly under Western opportunities, and whose scientific acquirements placed her high in rank among her peers in the college class, to accept again the position awarded her by the Code of Manu [The Code of Manu was a set of rules created by a scholar called Manu, which stated that women should accept a subservient position, always looked after by their fathers, husbands and sons].'[92]

The Prodigal Returns

In 1886, when Anandabai graduated, everything that she had worked so hard for seemed to be finally within her grasp. The diwan of Kolhapur offered Anandibai the post of a 'lady doctor' in Kolhapur. Her salary was to be 300 rupees per month, a good sum for the time, and her duties were to be in charge of the Albert Edward Hospital and instruct a class of girls in medicine. The diwan took care to specify Anandibai's duties. 'Mrs Joshi seems to think that we mean our pupils to be nurses only. Our object is much higher: to enable them to be general practitioners.'[93] This seems to be the first case where women were recruited to be doctors, not nurses.

Anandibai accepted the position. In her response, she wrote, 'Our Shasters [shastras (the holy texts of Hinduism)] require us to impart the gifts of healing without pay, and to this practice I shall adhere, but if I ever meant to take a fee from any one, it would assuredly be from those who are rich and powerful, and never from those who are poor and depressed.'[94]

This lofty dream was not to be. Anandibai's health had been delicate ever since the loss of her son. The harsh Philadelphia winters made it worse. The doctors prescribed meat and broth for her constant cough, but she refused to take those, to the consternation of her Western friends. Nutritious vegetarian food was not to be had easily. On the long voyage back to India, accompanied by Gopalrao, once again she struggled to find vegetarian food, making her even weaker.

Gopalrao had feared that priests would ostracise them for crossing the sea, but this fear, happily, did not come to pass. Anandibai was welcomed back in Bombay by those who were eager to mould her into an icon of Hindu womanhood. Chief amongst these, of course, was Tilak's English paper, *The Mahratta*, which welcomed the 'plucky pair', and praised Anandibai's costume, diet and habits.

There were numerous soirees and meetings to celebrate her triumphant return, but her health got steadily worse. For all her training in Western medicine, she was inexplicably treated by Ayurvedic doctors. There was panic as Gopalrao ran from place to place, trying to find a medical solution, all in vain. Finally, on 26 February 1887, twenty-two years old, she died. Her last words, according to Healey Dall, were, 'I have done all I could.'[95] In death, Anandibai once again bridged two countries. Her ashes would be taken by the Carpenters and interred in Poughkeepsie, New York, of all unlikely places. Her gravestone reads, 'First Brahmin woman to leave India to obtain an education.'[96]

Legacy: Role Model, But Also Perfect Wife

After her untimely death, Anandibai was mostly painted as a creation of Gopalrao, a woman who had been guided every step of the way by a benevolent husband. Her wifely devotion and adherence to Hindu customs was much praised. 'Although Anandibai was so young, her perseverance, undaunted courage and devotion to her husband were unparalleled,' wrote the *Dnyana Chakshu* paper.[97] There were also, of course, many references to her exalted higher caste. Meanwhile, *Kesari* made an unprecedented concession towards professional women in its editorial. 'It is indeed wonderful that a Brahman lady has proved to the world that the great qualities—perseverance, unselfishness, undaunted courage and an eager desire to serve one's country—do exist in the so-called weaker sex.'[98] *Kesari* then urged that Anandibai's memory be preserved by giving financial aid to another lady student of medicine. For a conservative paper, this was a huge step forward.

However, there were also those who criticised her trip to the US. The *Native Opinion* argued, 'Being no admirers of entrusting the education of our women to strangers in strange lands we may not be wrong in looking upon this sad event as one cumulative fatal result of foreign residence and its attendant wants, discomforts, and hard study.'[99] Meanwhile, back in Philadelphia, her shocked friends were inclined to blame Gopalrao—and the struggle to be a good Manuwadi wife—for her death.

If Anandibai had only known it, she was to serve as an exemplar for other women to follow. In 1892, Gurubai Karmakar became the second Indian woman to graduate in medicine from the WMC. Gurubai was a Christian, aided by missionaries. She eventually returned to India and worked at the American Marathi Mission in Bombay, helping cure leprosy patients.

But Anandibai's determination to be a good Hindu wife would be used as a weapon against those who followed, especially those who were not upper caste. In the years to come, Tilak and other Hindu conservatives would savagely criticise the maverick Rukhmabai Raut for not living up to the standards that Anandibai had set. No one would be quite good enough to measure up to the martyred Anandibai.

Gopalrao: The Merry Widower

After Anandibai's death, Gopalrao spent some time possibly steeped in regret over his behaviour, which had likely added to Anandibai's stress and mental trauma. In a letter to a friend, he mused, 'I wonder if she would not be living still, if I had never gone to America?'[100]

This uncharacteristic introspection did not last long, however. He revived rapidly, and made a very merry widower. He began to think again of how to revive his eccentric image. In October 1890, Gopalrao hosted a controversial tea party in Pune. The guests did not throw tea into the harbour like the famous guests at the Boston Tea Party, but they got into hot water, nevertheless. The venue was the spectacular Romanesque church of the Panch Haud mission, and the menu was 'Christian fare'—tea and biscuits—served by missionaries. The guest list comprised Pune's conservative Brahmins including Tilak and B.K. Gokhale, as well as fiery progressive reformers like B.G. Ranade and G.V. Kanitkar, who by then had already spoken out in support of widow remarriage and anti-caste movements. At the time, Pune was a bastion of Brahminism. Drinking tea offered by Christian missionaries was considered a sin for Brahmins, and a likely cause for excommunication.[101]

So why did Gopalrao organise this tea party? He probably wanted to bring the warring factions together, as well as bolster his own reputation as a reformer. It did not work out that way. Gopalrao, clearly intending to provoke, published the list of guests in the conservative paper *Pune Vaibhav*, insinuating that the reformers had won over the conservatives to their side.

Given the venue and the menu, there was a loud outcry from the conservative section, and Tilak and Gokhale had to defend their presence at the event. The conservatives were forced to refer the matter to the Shankaracharya (the religious title used by the head of a monastery), who appointed a committee of ten traditional shastris (a shastri is someone who teaches the shastras or religious texts) to investigate.

Tilak wriggled out of any punishment by claiming he had made a trip to Varanasi. Ranade refused to perform any penance, but eventually had to capitulate. Both the reformers and the conservatives were criticised for attending the event in each other's company. Gopalrao became a pariah in Pune society for his part in the whole messy affair, not that he cared greatly.

Gopalrao would go on to embarrass himself in more ways than one. In 1891, he would organise a ceremony in which a male and female donkey were 'married', in an attempt to criticise the marriage of old men to young women. He would attack those who had helped him in the past.

But his chief attention-seeking move was his conversion to Christianity, and then his reconversion to Hinduism after forty days. 'On 29 June 1891 he was "baptised and admitted into the Christian faith" by the Reverend Mr Taylor in a public ceremony at the famous spot known as the Sangam, the confluence of Pune's two rivers, as reported by *The Mahratta* on 5 July 1891. Very cannily, Gopalrao kept one foot in the Hindu Brahmin camp even after his "conversion" by continuing to wear his sacred thread and the sandalwood caste mark on his forehead. The somewhat predictable culmination of all this was his equally well-publicised and sensational "reconversion" after about forty days, claiming that he had never ceased to be a Hindu Brahmin. Through this entire spectacle, *The Mahratta* (which had mounted a strong attack on Ramabai after her conversion) as well as Pune Brahmins continued to treat him indulgently,' wrote Meera Kosambi.[102]

Gopalrao would die in Nasik in 1922, poor and largely deserted by friends and family weary of his eccentric ways. His pioneering young wife had been dead for thirty-five years by then. He too would leave a trail of confused biographers in his wake. Some, like Healey Dall, would be violently critical of his domineering ways, others, like the gushing Marathi press, would credit Anandibai's achievements entirely to her controlling husband. Like his wife, Gopalrao was complicated and often inscrutable. Unlike her, his name would soon be forgotten. He would never get the attention he yearned for.

CHAPTER THREE

The Working Mom

Kadambini Ganguly

'No opportunity has yet been offered to Indian medical women to show whether they are capable of taking responsible charge of large and important hospitals. Without giving those opportunities, it is not fair to pronounce that they are not competent to hold first class appointments.'

In 1891, the conservative *Bangabasi* paper departed from its usual subjects to call Kadambini Ganguly—a matronly lady doctor—a whore.

Kadambini was a mother of eight, a lover of embroidery and the caretaker for her elderly husband. All that mattered, though, was that she was the first Indian woman to actually practise as a doctor. This made her a perfect target for conservatives.

Anandibai was the first Indian woman to get a degree in medicine, but her early death deprived her of being the first Indian woman to practise medicine. When the film-maker Anant Mahadevan made a film about the fiery Rukhmabai Raut in 2016 and billed it as a movie about India's first practising doctor, there was outrage from some in the Bengali community. Why? Because Kadambini Ganguly—a quiet, low-profile, unsung Bengali doctor—was the first to merit the title. Many books have been written about her in Bengali, but she is not well-known outside the state.

Kadambini did not have a romantic death like Anandibai's, or a dramatic story like Rukhmabai's. Yet, in her own discreet, hardworking way, she was a pioneer. She was the first Indian woman graduate, along with Chandramukhi Bose. She went on to persuade the Calcutta Medical College to admit women students of medicine. She challenged entrenched British prejudice against Indian women doctors and went head-to-head with British colonialism—and won, even winning Florence Nightingale to her side.

And she did all this while caring for eight children—the ultimate working mother.

The Bengali Renaissance

Like Anandibai, Kadambini was certainly helped by the circumstances of her birth and her marriage. She was lucky to be born at the time of the Bengali Renaissance—a sweeping reformist movement spearheaded by the Brahmo Samaj, which broke conventions of marriage, education, dowry and the role of women. The Brahmo Samaj was founded by the reformer Raja Ram Mohan Roy, and continued by Debendranath Tagore, the patriarch of the Tagore family. It would foster some of India's most famous scientists, writers, poets, reformers and politicians. Most Brahmos were wealthy, anglicised, liberal Bengalis who worked alongside the British as professors, judges, civil servants and governors. Among the better-known Brahmos were Jagdish Chandra Bose, Rabindranath Tagore and P.C. Mahalanobis, the chairman of the first Planning Commission.

Kadambini was born in 1862 in Bhagalpur, Bihar, to Brajkishore Basu, a headmaster and stalwart of the Brahmo movement. The Brahmos were progressives, yet they were divided over the type of education to be given to women. Like her Victorian counterpart, the bhadramahila—the Bengali gentlewoman—was supposed to be educated, but not so educated that she forgot her place.

In 1871, Keshub Chandra Sen, a long-time member of the Brahmo movement, began a school called The Native Ladies Normal and Adult School. Sen, like many other men of the time, did not believe in teaching subjects like mathematics and science to women. Wrote Sen, 'Our chief aim is to organise a system of education specially adapted to the female mind and calculated to fit women for her position in society. The development of the true type of Hindu female character upon a plan of teaching at once natural and national is the primary subject of the undertaking.'[103] Thus, even amongst the Brahmos, the emphasis was often on grooming what they thought were perfect Hindu women, while the men were allowed to study whatever they wanted.

Education For Bengali Women: Memsahibs Or Bhadramahilas?

Luckily, there were a fringe of Brahmos who felt differently, which included Kadambini's father and his close friend, Durgamohan Das. In 1873, they partnered with a British woman, Annette Ackroyd, to start a school that propagated equality of the sexes. It was called the Hindu Mahila Vidyalaya (Hindu School for Girls) and was a game changer for a whole generation of Bengali women. The school, which Kadambini attended, taught maths, science, English, history, music and needlework. The girls were made to speak English during school hours, something that would shape Kadambini's future.

At the very same school taught a certain Dwarkanath Ganguly, a young man obsessively devoted to the education of women. He had radical ideas on this subject. Their paths would cross in the future; but for the moment he was only her teacher.

Ackroyd left the school in 1876, but it continued as the Banga Mahila Vidyalaya.

Kadambini aspired to continue her education upon graduation and to do this, she had to become a trailblazer, whether she so intended or not. To begin with, she and another female peer, Sarala Das, had to obtain a special dispensation from the University of Calcutta to appear at the entrance examination for admission, the first time women were allowed to give the same examination as men, albeit in a separate room.

Kadambini's liberal parents supported her, which was very unusual even amongst the Brahmos. It was one thing to preach against child marriage, another to actually educate daughters, and parents would withdraw their girls from school to marry them off. Indeed, Keshub Chandra Sen would marry his own daughter, Suniti, off to the maharajá of Cooch Behar when she was only fourteen, drawing harsh criticism from his followers.

Kadambini passed the entrance examination with merit, missing the first division by a single mark, and astonished the university by getting the second-highest marks in science. In those days, women were presumed to be terrible at science and maths, and more suited to cookery or needlework. This fact was remarked on by Alexander Arbuthnot, the vice chancellor of Calcutta university, who—while delivering the convocation address—said, 'Even in the exact sciences, a subject not exactly considered to be congenial to the female intellect— the young lady acquitted herself very credibly.'[104] But there was no provision for higher education for women. Here the famous Bethune School would play a pivotal role for Kadambini.

The Bethune School (originally the Calcutta Female School) was founded in 1849 with twenty-one girls by John Drinkwater Bethune, a member in the governor-general's council. There had been attempts to educate Bengali women before, by both missionaries and native Bengalis, such as Radhakanta Deb and Raja Ram Mohan Roy. However, missionary schools were regarded suspiciously by Hindu gentry, because the girls were mostly educated in Bible teachings. Bethune had different ideas. At the inauguration of the school, he reassured parents that the religion of their children 'would not be meddled with'. The girls were to be taught in Bengali, and English would be resorted to only occasionally. The school was called the

Calcutta Female School; talk of naming it after Queen Victoria was hastily squashed because it would deter Hindu parents.

Bethune died prematurely in 1851, and the managing committee decided Hindu involvement was needed. The man they decided to bring in had already distinguished himself in female education and social reform: Ishwar Chandra Vidyasagar, who became the secretary to the managing committee. By 1856, the girls were being taught reading, writing, maths, natural science, geography and, of course, the ever-present needlework. It would later merge with the Banga Mahila Vidyalaya in the 1870s as the government decided to take charge of the education of girls.

Seeing Kadambini's plight, the Bethune School decided to recruit new teachers to teach her college-level classes, and thus became the Bethune College.

Kadambini was awarded a scholarship of 15 rupees per month, a large sum in those days. Because of her unexpected success, the government also decided to award similar scholarships to three female candidates every year.

She would go on to greater things. Kadambini passed the First Arts examination from Bethune in 1880; not a degree, but still further than any woman had gone before. By this stage, she had begun to entertain the idea of pursuing medicine. There is no record of how or when this thought first struck her. The Calcutta Medical College (CMC), however, would not take women, so Kadambini tried a 'workaround': she decided to do a BA, a more advanced degree than the First Arts, which would guarantee admission into the medical college.

This too was not easy. Once again, the government scrambled to put the infrastructure into place, hiring teachers and increasing budgets. In 1882, Kadambini passed her BA from Bethune College and became one of the first women graduates in Bengal, along with Chandramukhi Bose. Their success was much celebrated. Bethune's support for the two women was particularly noteworthy, given Oxford only allowed women to graduate with a full degree in 1920 (though women were allowed to attend lectures).

Still, there was public censure. The conservative poet Ishwar Chandra Gupta wrote disparagingly about the new breed of educated Bengali women; many shared his views. A rough translation of his poem goes:

> All our lassies, smacking their fingers and books in their
> hands will spiral down to infamy;
> With knowledge of 'A, B' and dressed like memsahibs, and
> surely muttering in their foreign lingo;
> Wait a few more days, my brothers, surely you will not miss
> the sight;
> Of them driving their own carriages to Gorer Math (the
> Calcutta Maidan) for unrestricted fun and frolic.[105]

But the Brahmos ignored these mutterings and continued to try and get more girls educated. In 1888, the Bethune School had 136 students—eighty-seven Brahmos, forty-four Hindus and five Christians.[106]

Then came the final hurdle: the medical degree. Kadambini's BA did not win her admission to the CMC. The Bengali papers came to her support. Even before Kadambini came along, the *Brahmo Public Opinion*, the newspaper of the Brahmo movement, had been outspoken in supporting the entry of women into medical colleges. 'The want of good female doctors is very keenly felt in Bengal, and we presume other parts of India too...' it said in an 1878 editorial. 'We know of several instances in orthodox Hindu families, where the female members suffer from the most complicated diseases but yet would not allow male doctors to visit and treat them. The consequence is that they are treated second hand through the assistance of uneducated quack native midwives and in ninety-nine cases out of a hundred, are never radically cured.'[107] The newspaper went on to call for the breaking of social rules, and the tearing down of the zenana, supported by other newspapers.

But before Kadambini could take on the medical colleges, she did something few could have predicted for the bright young woman who had all of Calcutta curious.

Marriage To A Mentor

On 12 January 1883, Kadambini married her friend, philosopher and guide, Dwarkanath Ganguly. She was twenty-one, her groom a widower who was already thirty-nine and with three children of his own.

Many in the Brahmo movement were shocked at the marriage, perhaps because they believed being married would hinder her, or perhaps because of the huge age difference. Another Bengali woman, Abala Das, had dropped out of her medical course at the Madras Medical College after her marriage to the biologist Jagdish Chandra Bose, and many well-wishers feared that Kadambini too would be swallowed by domestic responsibilities. Several of Dwarkanath's friends refused to attend the marriage.

At the wedding, the age difference between them was even more apparent. A local Brahmo newspaper editor was so moved by the young Kadambini's dewy beauty that he wrote a flowery poem, borrowing a verse from Wordsworth:

> She was Phantom of delight
> When first she gleaned upon my Sight
> A lovely apparition sent to be a moment's Ornament
> Her eyes as stars of Twilight.[108]

Dwarkanath, like many of the Brahmo movement, was in favour of Indian women receiving higher education in general and becoming doctors in particular. But there was a strong puritan streak in the otherwise progressive Brahmo movement. The objective of this was to make women better wives and mothers, and also to discourage husbands from a life of vice—visiting prostitutes, drinking and smoking.

The Brahmos believed that husbands and wives should have shared interests, which—given how uneducated most Indian women were—was almost impossible at that time. An article titled 'Ardhangini' in the *Bamabodhini Patrika*, stated,

'When the husband is busy determining the distance between the sun and other constellations, the wife is busy measuring the dimensions of her pillowcases. When the husband thinks about the stars and planets in the sky, the wife is then at the kitchen, determining the reflexes and speed of the cook.'[109]

The idea of a woman being educated for her own sake—not to be more interesting and a better companion to her husband—was apparently too radical to contemplate. Still, this was as progressive as women could hope for at the time, and more so than the rest of India.

Later, Kadambini and Dwarkanath's unusual and mutually supportive marriage would win much praise. The American historian David Kopf wrote of the couple, 'Ganguli's wife, Kadambini, was appropriately enough the most accomplished and liberated Brahmo woman of her time. From all accounts, their relationship was most unusual in being founded on mutual love, sensitivity and intelligence. Mrs. Ganguli's case was hardly typical even among the more emancipated Brahmo and Christian women in contemporary Bengali society. Her ability to rise above circumstances and to realize her potential as a human being made her a prize attraction to Sadharan Brahmos dedicated ideologically to the liberation of Bengal's women.'[110]

Kadambini never wrote about her marriage, or indeed about anything else, so it is hard to know what she thought. But Dwarkanath certainly supported Kadambini through her various battles. 'Her life was very different from that of Rukhmabai or Anandibai. She got constant support from her father from childhood days, and in her later life her husband Dwarkanath became her mentor, her friend, her philosopher and her guide,' agrees historian and author Mousumi Bandyopadhyay Majumdar.[111]

In this, Kadambini was incredibly lucky, given the terrible, often abusive marriages of her peers. 'Whatever reference we get about their conjugal life gives the picture of... a compatible life and it is obvious that a perfect understanding and balance existed between them. Both of them were respectful to each other,' says Majumdar.[112]

Kadambini Versus The Calcutta Medical College

Soon after her marriage, Kadambini began her battle with the CMC, a move that was to pave the way for dozens of women medical students in the years to come.

The CMC had been founded by Lord William Bentinck in 1835 and had a history of breaking convention. It had been established on the recommendation of a committee set up by the East India Company, which regarded the training of Calcutta medical professionals, especially native Indians, as inadequate.

A key figure behind the CMC was Madhusudan Gupta, a physician who began life as an Ayurvedic doctor and Sanskrit scholar. Gupta rapidly became a supporter of practical anatomy and dissections. At the time, Hindu customs and religious taboos prohibited the touching of dead bodies. Gupta, undeterred, gathered support from Sanskrit and Ayurveda literature, including the ancient physician Susruta, to argue that dissection was allowed. Still, the procuring of a body was a challenge, as the Hindu community continued to oppose dissections, and Hindu priests kept vigil outside the college to stop bodies from being brought in. In 1836, Gupta dissected a dead body on his own, the first Indian trained in Western medicine to do so, encouraged by none other than John Drinkwater Bethune.

This, then, was the path-breaking institution that Kadambini was trying to enter. Pioneering though it was, entry was still barred for women.

Despite the backing Kadambini received from editorials in Bengali newspapers, especially women's ones, and the Brahmo movement, a considerable hurdle stood in her way. The acting principal of the CMC, R. Harvey, was against female students for several reasons. In June 1882, Harvey wrote a letter in which he called mixed classes 'objectionable and likely to exercise a demoralising influence upon the students of both sexes'. He suggested a separate school be set up. Harvey also believed that 'there does not exist among the native community a general demand for female physicians and nurses, and that more extended training in midwifery would be sufficient.'[113]

Other members of the Indian Medical Council also agreed that Indian women were deeply unfit for the study of medicine. Even if they were fit, they contended, the Indian community would never, ever entertain female doctors.

Once again, the *Brahmo Public Opinion* leapt in to defend women doctors, citing the case of Abala Bose, who had had to travel all the way to Madras to get a medical education. The general public also put pressure on the government. Finally, the lieutenant general of Bengal, Augustus Rivers Thompson, stepped in.

Thompson was ahead of his time in judging that what had worked in Europe, and in Madras, could work in the rest of India. 'The aptitude of women for the study of medicine is no longer open to discussion and doubt,' he wrote firmly. 'For his own part, the Lieutenant-General looks forward to a not distant time when Calcutta hospitals shall be partly officered by lady doctors.' The news was broadly welcomed by the press and public, but the pressure on Kadambini to do well must have been intense.

Kadambini entered the college in June 1883. No record survives of her college years, or how she managed in a class filled with men.

We can assume that it was extremely difficult. And a crushing blow was to come. In 1886, she appeared in her final exams, but failed to graduate by just one mark, in the subjects of materia medica and anatomy. She could not get an MB (Bachelor of Medicine) degree. Thousands of miles away, Anandibai Joshi had just qualified at the Women's Medical College in Pennsylvania.

Kadambini's son, Prabhat Chandra Gangopadhyay, was later to allege that the examiner, Dr R.C. Chandra, failed her deliberately because he resented her success. Kadambini could have re-sat the exams, but she did not, for reasons best known to her.

Instead, she was awarded a GBMC (Graduate of Bengal Medical College), a lesser qualification, which nevertheless allowed her to practice. In 1888, she was appointed a doctor at the Lady Dufferin Women's Hospital, with a salary of 300 rupees per month. This was a good salary for the time.[114] Thus, while she did not have a full medical qualification, she was still the first Indian woman doctor to practise in India.

Kadambini had an unlikely supporter when she graduated: Florence Nightingale, who seemed to have changed her mind about women doctors since the days of Elizabeth Blackwell. In February 1888, she wrote to a friend, 'Do you know or could tell me anything about Mrs Ganguly, or give me any advice? This young lady married after she made up her mind to become a doctor and has had one, if not two children since. But she was absent only thirteen days for her lying in and did not miss a single lecture.'[115] Nightingale wrote that she had been asked to recommend Kadambini for posts in Calcutta.

However, it was one thing to practice, it was another to actually attract patients. In 1888, Kadambini placed advertisements in *The Hindu Patriot* and *The Bengalee*. They read:

A Card

Mrs Ganguly BA

45-5 Beniatola Lane, College Square North East Corner

Calcutta

Having studied in the Medical College for five years and obtained a college diploma to study medicine, surgery and midwifery, has commenced practice and treats women and children. Consultation free for poor patients at her home between 2 and 3 pm daily.[116]

Apart from the reluctance of patients to consult a lady doctor, Kadambini ran into another obstacle. The enemy this time was a formidable one: British colonialism and prejudice. And it came from a source that was meant to help, but only hindered.

The Dufferin Fund: Godsend Or Colonial Legacy?

When Lady Harriet Dufferin, wife of the then viceroy, was leaving for India in 1884, Queen Victoria asked her to start a scheme for women's medical education. Thus, the Countess of Dufferin Fund was set up in 1885, aiming to improve women's healthcare. At its inception, Lord Dufferin said, 'Our ambition is to furnish every district, however remote, with a supply of highly trained female doctors, at all events, with nurses, midwives and female medical assistants.' But the Dufferin Fund, though it meant well, had a major flaw: it favoured European women doctors over natives. By 1885, more and more British women had begun to study medicine in the UK, but on graduating, they found nobody would give them jobs, preferring instead to hire men. India thus became a massive market for British women doctors who desperately needed jobs, having spent much of their savings on getting their degrees.

Thus, nearly all the lady doctors of the first grade (those who were paid higher salaries and given more responsibility) were European, while the Indians worked as hospital assistants under them, and provided cheap labour. As admitted by the Dufferin Fund itself, the European women were clever, but had no knowledge of native ways and customs. Wrote *The Bengalee*, 'The appointments have practically become a close preserve for European and Eurasian lady doctors, and Indian ladies are systematically kept out.'[117] By 1887, there were about 150 Indian women enrolled in medical programmes under the Dufferin Fund, but crucially, doctors educated in England were paid 450 rupees per month, while local hospital assistants were paid 50 rupees per month.[118]

The other flawed principle that the Dufferin Fund was founded on was the imperialist idea of zenana medical care. Right from the start, the idea took root that Indian women would not go to male doctors, or even leave the house, because they were secluded in the zenana. The Dufferin Fund ignored the many Indian women, mostly lower caste or poor, who had no choice but to leave the house. By the 1880s, as the London School of Medicine was turning out British women doctors by the dozen, the zenana school of thought was commonplace. Even Sophia Jex-Blake, the grand doyenne of the University of Edinburgh, emphasised the need for medical women in India to attend patients in zenanas.

Why was this emphasis on the zenana problematic? Chiefly because it infantilised Indian women, who were thought to be so restricted that they could not train as doctors themselves, and ignored the steady trickle of Indian women who were eager to become doctors, especially those emerging from Bengal. Neither Anandibai nor Kadambini, for instance, were supported in their education by the Dufferin Fund.

Meanwhile, as the Dufferin Fund endured, it began to take on an increasingly evangelical tinge. The women doctors hired were often missionaries, who used medicine as a way to spread their gospel. Chief among these missionary doctors was the brilliant Mary Scharlieb, who was one of the first women graduates of the Madras Medical College. Scharlieb would go on to study at the London School of Medicine, teach in the gynaecology department of the Madras Medical College and work with Elizabeth Garrett Anderson. Scharlieb was a remarkable and tenacious woman who paved the way for many women doctors, but she was also an evangelical Christian who approvingly quoted Rudyard Kipling on the 'white man's burden'.

'Medical mission work indeed constitutes the most attractive exposition of the work and aims of the Good Physician, but it is also the foundation of the truly educative and statesmanlike endeavours which are meant to draw into one state ancient, spiritually-minded India, and the modern, materialistic West. Indeed it is in the humble mission compound, with its narrow means and its want of earthly prestige, that we find the nearest approximation to the spiritual gladness of the early Christian Church. Take up the White Man's Burden, the savage wars of peace, fill full the mouth of Famine, and bid the sickness cease,' wrote Scharlieb.[119]

While Scharlieb was incredibly qualified, many of the women missionaries were not. So poor was the quality of some of them that stalwarts of the movement, like Elizabeth Garrett Anderson and Sophia Jex-Blake, felt compelled to write to the papers, arguing against the wholesale export of unqualified women to India. According to Sophia, the Church of England Missionary Zenana Society was particularly at fault for disregarding 'professional skill'. There was also criticism that the European lady doctors were missionaries first and doctors second—hired to evangelise rather than heal.

Kadambini was one of the Indian doctors who were thus shortchanged. She was appointed as an officiating doctor with the Dufferin Fund, and was denied charge of a ward, the only way to acquire skills. Frustrated and offended, she wrote an open letter to a local newspaper. This is one of the few letters written by Kadambini that exist, and her anger at the injustice is apparent. She wrote, 'By the present arrangements, English medical women, though they may not at first possess higher qualifications than their Indian sisters, will soon acquire much better skills by performing hospital duties… No opportunity has yet been offered to Indian medical women to show whether they are capable of taking responsible charge of large and important hospitals. Without giving those opportunities to prove their capabilities, it is not fair to pronounce that they are not competent to hold first class appointments.'[120]

The 'Unchaste' Lady Doctor

Kadambini also had to contend with deep prejudice from conservative Hindus. This motherly woman, who worked at the Dufferin all day and took care of her large family in the evening, seemed still to be considered a threat to conservative Brahmos in particular, and to conservative men everywhere. In 1891, the *Bangabasi* called her a whore.[121]

Shortly afterwards, the *Indian Messenger* published an article arguing that giving women opportunities for education would make them unchaste and wayward. 'The maintenance of female virtue is incompatible with their liberty,' wrote the *Messenger*.[122]

Why did these journals make this ludicrous charge? Historian Malavika Karlekar explains: 'In calling Kadambini a whore, *Bangabasi* was externalising the male fear of a competitive and competent woman. Her status as a wife and mother was no defence against the conservative stance which felt that a career and life outside the home threatened traditional notions of chastity and femininity.'[123]

To his credit, Dwarkanath stepped forward quickly to defend Kadambini. He filed a suit for defamation against the *Bangabasi* editor Mahesh Chandra Pal, who was found guilty, fined 100 rupees and sentenced to six months imprisonment. After this, the *Indian Messenger* also later changed its tune, calling Kadambini a 'distinguished member of the medical profession'. But the incident showed how even marriage and a brood of children were no guarantee against sexist abuse.

A British Degree For Equal Treatment

After a few years of being treated as inferior to British doctors, Kadambini realised that perhaps only a British degree would bring her equal treatment. She travelled to Edinburgh in February 1893, to sit for the exams of the Royal College of Surgeons, leaving her children with her sister. Once again, she wrote nothing about the difficulties of this solo journey, or why she chose Edinburgh, although it is easy to speculate.

Apart from the Edinburgh Seven, the University of Edinburgh's medical school also had famous male graduates. Charles Darwin had entered the school, though he would leave with only a degree in biology. One of the most famous was Sir Arthur Conan Doyle, the creator of Sherlock Holmes, who studied medicine at the university from 1876 to 1881, only a decade or so before Kadambini. Doyle found inspiration for Holmes in Joseph Bell, a saturnine Scottish surgeon and teacher who was his mentor at the university.

Kadambini spent only a few months in Edinburgh. That was enough for her to accumulate several diplomas. She passed the triple qualification exam on 18 July 1893, the only woman of fourteen successful candidates that year. She was awarded three diplomas: the Licentiate of the Royal College of Physicians, Licentiate of the Royal College of Surgeons and Licentiate of the Faculty of Physicians and Surgeons. And by November 1893, she was back in Calcutta.

This time, she got her due. Bolstered by her foreign qualifications, she was appointed to the post she really wanted in Lady Dufferin Hospital, that of superintendent. By this time, public feeling towards lady doctors, even Bengali ones, had changed. Lady Dufferin wrote a glowing letter to Kadambini, in which she expressed her support and reassured her that qualified Indian women doctors would be considered with favour.[124]

Private Practice As A Working Mother

After a few years, Kadambini began a private practice of her own. Very little information survives of Kadambini's daily life. She seemed to write few letters, wrote no diary and generally kept a low profile. As possibly one of the first professional working mothers in her milieu, with a flourishing practice and eight children to take care of, her life was perhaps too busy to contemplate her legacy or rest on her laurels, unlike her less overburdened contemporaries.

'She was a working mom—mother of eight children, one of them being mentally challenged, and of course she used to have a very busy schedule, because apart from meeting her responsibilities as a doctor she was also engaged in other philanthropic activities and also in contemporary politics,' says Bandyopadhyay Majumdar. 'Indeed it is very frustrating that in the absence of any diary or memoirs we cannot draw a total picture of her life.'[125]

What does survive is a picture of a woman initially much sought after by the rich and famous. In 1895, Kadambini treated the queen mother of the royal family of Nepal, and apparently saved her life. In return, along with gifts of money and jewellery, she was given a pony, which her children and grandchildren greatly enjoyed playing with. However, Kadambini was also gradually becoming conscious of her social responsibility. She treated pardanashin women—women who observed rigid rules of seclusion—and would later join politics.

Despite her fame, Kadambini was often treated as no more than a midwife, or dai. One incident that clearly upset Kadambini and her family occurred when she was called to attend a childbirth in a rich family. The birth was difficult, and it was only because of her expertise that the mother and baby survived. Afterwards, Kadambini, to her great anger, was asked to eat her lunch with the maidservant, and then to clean the area. Kadambini's daughter was in tears when she saw that all her mother's learning would not prevent her from being called a dai.[126]

Entering Politics

In the late 1890s, Kadambini began to develop an interest in politics and the nationalist movement. Up until then, women had not been a part of the nationalist struggle. The bhadralok (the Bengali term for gentleman or well educated person) believed that the bhadramahila (the female equivalent) was incapable of or uninterested in understanding politics.

Decades later, when Mahatma Gandhi launched the Civil Disobedience movement, he asked women to join in and walk beside their men. 'The women of India should have as much share in winning Swaraj (the term used for independence for India) as the men. In this peaceful struggle women can out-distance men by many a mile,' he said. Jawaharlal Nehru agreed, and addressing women students at Allahabad in 1928, he said, 'The future of India cannot consist of dolls and playthings, and if you made half the population of the country a mere plaything of the other half, an encumbrance on others, how will you ever make progress?'[127]

At the time Kadambini became interested in politics, women were still a long way from being included. But the Brahmos were ahead of their time in most fields. To begin with, there were numerous ladies' associations which brought together both sexes for social gatherings, contrary to the practice of the more orthodox Hindus. This helped make the women more confident. Kadambini cut her teeth on these activities and learnt how to speak in public, organise events and mingle with men.

Once again, it was Dwarkanath who helped her enter the arena, by campaigning for women to attend Congress sessions. In the 1889 session of the Indian National Congress in Bombay, no less than ten women attended as delegates. But in that session, they were mere figureheads and not allowed to speak. After protests, this was remedied in the sixth session of the Indian National Congress. This session stated in its report, 'The dear ladies resented, and we think justly, the silence imposed upon them. They refused to recognise, as having any practical value, the aesthetic charm which their presence on the platform conferred on the entire gathering. They said: Better have some pretty wax figures, nicely dressed, on the platform, they will serve your purpose equally well.'[128]

A woman was thus allowed to speak in the sixth session in 1890, and that woman was Kadambini. Her speech was unremarkable in itself, merely proposing Pherozeshah Mehta for president, but broke new ground as the first made by a woman speaker from the Congress platform.

Dwarkanath died in 1898, and for some time Kadambini restricted her activities, perhaps in grief for the husband who had always stood by her.

In 1907, when Gandhi was imprisoned in South Africa, she took over and became the head of the Transvaal Indian Association, which helped Indians in that region. In 1922, she travelled to Bihar and Orissa to investigate the conditions of female workers in the coal mines, on behalf of an enquiry commission set up by the government.

Dying In The Harness

Death came suddenly for Kadambini, on 3 October 1923. She died on the job while attending an ailing patient. Her funeral costs were met out of the amount she received for her visit: 50 rupees. Until the end, she remained on her feet, tireless and independent.

The first Indian woman to become a practising doctor would fade into relative obscurity, and her name would be mostly forgotten for years. But the impact of her choices would endure, as Kadambini's dogged and low-profile success would inspire many Bengali women to go into medicine, and prompt colleges to make arrangements for them. In 1889, Bidhumukhi Bose and Virginia Mary Mitter graduated from the Calcutta Medical College, aided by scholarships of 20 rupees per month. A girls' hostel was built to accommodate the growing number of female students. Seats were reserved for women candidates, as it began to be slowly recognised that women doctors were a good thing for everyone.

Bethune College, which had groomed Kadambini, went on to produce many other women who took an active part in public life, including Pritilata Wadedar, a graduate of philosophy in 1928, who went on to become a fiery revolutionary and nationalist.

Kadaminini's stepdaughter, Jyotirmoyee Ganguly, would become a teacher and the first woman councillor of the Calcutta Corporation. Perhaps inspired by Kadambini, Jyotirmoyee was active in politics and the Satyagraha movement, and was imprisoned twice. She would meet an untimely death by police firing on 22 November 1945, while taking out a street protest.

In the last few years, Kadambini's name has become more familiar. Calcutta Medical College named a neonatal medical ward after her. In February 2020, two TV Bengali TV shows based on Kadambini's life were announced, one called *Prathama Kadambini*, starring Ushashi Roy on Zee Jalsa, the other called *Kadambini*, starring Solanki Roy.

One preview showed a wide-eyed, apprehensive Kadambini entering a home. 'Where is the doctor? This is a woman,' shouts a shocked lady of the home. Kadambini remains unperturbed, walking sedately through the house carrying her large doctor's bag. *'Rogi kothay?'* she asks, calmly. (Where is the patient?) Bemused and with their mouths hanging open, the household shows her to the patient. And with that small gesture of recognition over 150 years ago, lady doctors and working mothers crossed the threshold into acceptance.

CHAPTER FOUR

The Rule Breaker

Rukhmabai Raut

'*Men cannot, in the least, understand the wretchedness which we Hindu women have to endure. Because you cannot enter our feelings, do not think that we are satisfied with the life of drudgery that we live, and that we have no taste for an aspiration after a higher life.*'

It is March 1887. A young woman stands in a Mumbai court room, facing the husband she despises. Shortly, a judge is going to pronounce on whether a Hindu wife can break the sacrament of a child marriage. She is twenty-two, but she has never lived with her husband, and never wants to.

The judge rules that the woman must live with her husband or go to jail for six months. But this is not the end. Instead, it is the start of a long, bitter battle by a woman who wanted to study to be a proud doctor, not an unwilling wife. She would become the first Hindu woman to do the unthinkable: leave her husband and seek a divorce.

The woman was Rukhmabai Raut (sometimes spelt Rakhmabai), a woman from a historically oppressed caste who was to smash every rule of Hindu society. If Anandibai was one facet of Indian women—the comforting face of tradition—the radical Rukhmabai Raut was the polar opposite. At the very time that Anandibai and Kadambini were supported by husbands, Rukhmabai was trying to get rid of hers.

Rukhmabai would cause a yawning chasm in Hindu society,

between liberals who supported women's education and the conservatives who bitterly opposed it. She would be instrumental in the passage of a law that raised the age of consent for child marriages. She would be savagely attacked and shamed by Bal Gangadhar Tilak and other upper-caste Hindu conservatives, who wanted Swaraj, but not for women, and especially not for lower-caste women.

Rukhmabai did not write an autobiography. She also burnt most of the letters she received at the end of every month from well-wishers and supporters, possibly to erase painful memories.[129] We thus have only a fragmented image of her. What impressions we have, though, are more vivid and revelatory than the narratives surrounding any other lady doctor.

Dr Sakharam Arjun: Father, Teacher, Visionary

Rukhmabai was born in Bombay in 1864, to Jayantibai and Janardan Pandurang. When she was two, her father died. At the time, her mother was only seventeen. Jayantibai belonged to the Suthar or carpenter caste. Unlike upper castes, the Suthars allowed the remarriage of widows. Six years later, her mother married Dr Sakharam Arjun, a prominent doctor, botanist and reformer, who was also a widower. Jayantibai had property of her own through her first husband, a fact that would later become significant.

Dr Sakharam was an intriguing figure. He taught at Grant Medical College and was one of the two original founders of the Bombay Natural History Society. He conducted a number of studies on the uses of plants and would later write a catalogue of Indian medicinal plants. Rukhmabai would be deeply influenced by her stepfather's liberal ways.

Nevertheless, even Dr Sakharam was not powerful enough to defy Hindu custom and stop Rukhmabai being married off as a child. At eleven, she was married to Dadaji Bhikaji, a poor relative of Dr Sakharam's, who was nineteen. It was agreed that Rukhmabai would join her husband after she attained puberty. Dr Sakharam was uncomfortable with the marriage. Later, he would participate in efforts to reform Hindu customs, and would speak passionately in favour of separating Hindu law from Hindu custom. Dr Sakharam would also go on to recommend that young children betrothed in marriage should have the chance to 'ratify' the marriage once older. This was a radical thought for the time, and one can see how Rukhmabai might have idolised this unusual, charismatic man.

At eleven, Rukhmabai had already attained puberty, after which girls were traditionally expected to go to their husband's house to consummate the marriage. But Dr Sakharam refused to send her. To begin with, he thought she was too young. Later he developed further misgivings. Dadaji had grown into a drunken and dissipated man, with a string of unpaid debts. He was greatly influenced by his uncle, Narayan Dhurmaji, with whom he lived. Dhurmaji was a dissolute man with several mistresses. Rukhmabai began to feel a deep aversion for them both, and over the next few years, avoided all contact with her husband, aided by her sympathetic stepfather.

Rukhmabai writes, 'I was married on conditions that he should be thoroughly provided by us, but that he should study and become a good man. However, in a few months after the marriage he began to neglect his duties, leaving the school and disobeying my father and grandfather, fell into bad companies (sic).'[130]

Dr Sakharam became a key figure in young Rukhmabai's life. He mingled with reformers and liberals, both Indian and European, and Rukhmabai learnt much from them, including English. One of the visitors was Vishnu Shastri Pandit, a fervent supporter of women's education. In such company, it is hardly surprising that Rukhmabai began to do the most dangerous of things for a woman of that time: think for herself. 'I had a great liking for study while a great disgust for married life, and though not fortunate enough to attain school after the age of 11 years I began to learn English at home, after leaving the school. I used to ask a number of pronunciations and meanings of

English words at a time whenever my European lady friends happened to call. I began seriously to consider the former and present condition of our Hindu women, and wished to do something if in our power to ameliorate our present sufferings,' wrote Rukhmabai.[131]

Rukhmabai was no good Hindu wife. She was a flouter of convention, a breaker of rules, a rebel with a cause. Right from childhood, she was certain that her early marriage had stopped her from achieving everything she wanted.

The Suit

Eventually, in March 1884, when Rukhmabai was twenty, Dadaji grew tired of waiting. He sent a legal notice to Sakharam, asking that she be allowed to come and live with him. It is likely that Dadaji may have been at least partly motivated by Rukhmabai's money. She owned a substantial amount of property, though the amount was in dispute. (Some accounts estimate it at being 25,000 rupees—a huge sum in those days. Rukhmabai estimated it at half the amount.)

Dr Sakharam was in a dilemma. He replied that Rakhmabai was only living in his house because of Dadaji's strained finances. He ended with a sarcastic aside. 'I have not the slightest wish to detain her even now and I shall be glad if your client provides her with a suitable house and takes her away, which is however his own look-out.'[132]

Reading between the lines, Dr Sakharam was walking a tightrope. By this juncture, he knew his ward's dislike for her husband, and was determined to keep her with him. So, he had to come up with a plausible excuse while he thought about his next move. Unfortunately, he had less time than he thought.[133]

On 25 March, a party of people went to bring the reluctant bride to Dadaji, including Narayan Dhurmaji, Dadaji's elder brother and a solicitor's clerk. Rukhmabai refused to go with them. Initially, her objections were fairly elementary. First, she argued that Dadaji had no proper house for her, and that he would have to rent another house.

Then, through her solicitors, she argued that he was in a poor state of health. Both parties knew what the real truth was.

A humiliated Dadaji filed a suit and brought counter-charges of his own. His contention was that the real reason for Rukhmabai not joining him was the pressure brought upon her by her mother and her maternal grandfather, who wanted to keep her property within the family. Rukhmabai dismissed these charges, arguing that the value of the property was half what he had cited, and that her mother and grandfather were not the covetous, grasping people that Dadaji alleged.

But even as Rukhmabai was responding to these petty charges, she was moving firmly, inexorably, towards a revolutionary position, which must have frightened even her. In her reply to Dadaji's plaint, she argued that, as she was too young to give consent to the marriage, she could not be bound to it. This was essentially an attack on the entire Hindu family system, the custom of child marriage and the concept of marriage as a sacred union. It was one woman against the might of the Hindu sacrament.

Dr Sakharam now had to decide whether or not to support his fiery ward. It was not an easy decision. It was one thing to argue that Dadaji was unable to maintain Rukhmabai in the style to which she was accustomed. It was another, entirely, to take on Hindu custom. It is to Dr Sakharam's great credit that he came down on Rukhmabai's side, despite criticism from his caste elders. However, Rukhmabai would eventually have to fight the battle on her own—Dr Sakharam would die only months before the suit came to court.

The Letters

Rukhmabai followed up her legal response with two letters in *The Times of India*, written under the pseudonym 'A Hindoo Lady'. The letters were deeply shocking for their time and created a great stir.

Rukhmabai was lucky in that the editor of *The Times of India* at the time was a British man called Henry Curwen.

With his eye for a good story, Curwen immediately recognised the letters for what they were: the nineteenth-century version of click-bait, guaranteed to enrage and fascinate readers. He wrote an editorial recommending that readers view the letters as the true and authentic protest of a Hindu lady against injustice.

The letters savagely criticised child marriage. Wrote Rukhmabai in the first letter, 'Marriage does not impose any insuperable obstacle on men in the course of their studies... If married early they are not called upon to go to the house, and to submit to the tender mercies of a mother-in-law, nor is any restraint put upon their actions because of their marriage.'[134]

She went on to describe the completely different plight of women, 'But the case with women is the very reverse of this. If the girl is married at the age of eight (as most of them are), her parents are at liberty to send her to school till she is ten years old; but, if they wish to continue her at school longer, they must obtain the express permission of the girl's mother-in-law.[135]

'Thus, Mr. Editor, when we are just beginning to appreciate education, we are taken away from school... For even a girl, who is so exceptionally blessed as to have parents holding the most liberal views on education, can only prosecute her studies for three or four years longer, for she is generally a mother before she is 14, when she must of sheer necessity give up the dream of mental cultivation, and face the hard realities of life.'[136]

Rukhmabai wrote about her own dream to study and explore the world. 'Sir, I am one of those unfortunate Hindu women, whose hard lot it is to suffer the unnameable miseries entailed by the custom of early marriage. This wicked practice has destroyed the happiness of my life. It comes between me and that thing which I prize above all others—study and mental cultivation.' She then bravely went on to call for intervention by the government, and suggest that the age of marriage be raised to fifteen for the bride and twenty for the groom, to root out 'the pernicious custom'.[137]

It is impossible to overestimate the impact of this passionate letter. Rukhmabai had lit a grenade under a cloistered, ossified Hindu society. No Hindu woman had dared to take on child marriage, except the maverick Pandita Ramabai, whose reception has been discussed in Chapter 2.

At the time, local custom believed that an unmarried girl over eleven or twelve, or past the age of puberty, would bring bad luck to the house. The Hindu shastras were considered sacrament and set in stone; even the British rulers would not meddle with them, for the sake of public order. It is true that Hindu reformers such as Raja Ram Mohan Roy and Ishwar Chandra Vidyasagar had begun criticising the shastras by this time, but for a Hindu woman to do it, particularly a lower-caste woman, was unthinkable.

Explains historian and author Sudhir Chandra, 'Rukhmabai's attack on early as well as infant marriage was radical for the time. There were many who condemned infant marriage, but considered early marriage shastric and essential to the Hindu domestic economy. Rukhmabai, in contrast, wanted no marriage to be legal unless the bride is fifteen and the bridegroom is twenty years old.'[138]

The Friend In Need: Behramji Malabari

Rukhmabai drew great support from an unlikely source: a Parsi poet, author and reformer called Behramji Malabari. Malabari was something of a Renaissance man and one of the most fascinating figures of the time. He wrote poetry in both Gujarati and English, and one of his works, *The Indian Muse*, was widely praised by William Wordsworth, Florence Nightingale and the Sanskrit scholar Max Müller.

In 1880, Malabari became the editor of the *Indian Spectator*, a tiny and struggling paper which he bought for 25 rupees. His aim was 'to make it the people of India's own paper'. By this time, many native papers had begun to report on the plight of India's child widows. Malabari was deeply affected, but as a Parsi, he was inclined to be cautious in criticising the hoary traditions of Hindu society.

Malabari believed that mere discussion of social evils without the support of the state was pointless. And thus, in August 1884, he published what he called his *Notes on Infant Marriage and Enforced Widowhood*, a pamphlet sent to 4,000 leading Englishmen and Hindus. The pamphlet was translated into many vernacular languages and widely circulated. The then viceroy Lord Ripon met with Malabari and promised to consider his arguments.

In the pamphlet, Malabari deplored the 'social evil' of 'baby marriage' and demanded laws to prevent it. Malabari did not go as far as Rukhmabai in demanding a minimum age of fifteen. He was only against infant marriages and favoured fixing the age at twelve.

But even so, Rukhmabai was cheered by the pamphlet. For the first time, she had support from influential, powerful men. 'I felt that fortune was about to smile on the unhappy daughters of India,' she wrote in her first letter.

Rukhmabai wrote a second letter in *The Times of India*. This time, the canny Curwen gave it even more coverage. The newspaper carried an editorial that praised Rukhmabai as a 'high spirited woman of refinement, culture and intellectual superiority... intimately acquainted with the position of her sisters in Europe'.[139]

Curwen was also smart enough to time the publication of the letters well. The first letter was published in June 1885, a few months before Rukhmabai's suit was to be heard. The second was published on 19 September 1885, on the exact day her case came up in the Bombay High Court.

This one was even more biting and brave, condemning smug Hindu patriarchy as no one had ever done before.

'Being men, the shastric law givers have painted themselves noble and pure, and have laid every conceivable sin and impurity at our door. If these worthies are to be trusted, we are a set of unclean animals, created by god for the special service and gratification of man, who by divine right can treat or maltreat us at his sweet will.'[140]

But Rukhmabai was not indifferent to the problems of young men coerced into marriage either. 'The poor fellow, hardly out of his teens, is saddled with a wife and a family of two or three children...'[141] Early marriage, she argued, hurt both men and women.

A Powerful Opponent:
Rukhmabai Makes An Enemy Of Bal Gangadhar Tilak

At around this time, Rukhmabai made a formidable foe: Bal Gangadhar Tilak. By the 1880s, Tilak had earned a reputation for being a fervent and much-vaunted nationalist, but also a stubborn conservative when it came to women and those from the lower castes.

Tilak was born to a Chitpavan Brahmin family in Ratnagiri and grew up in the orthodox society of Pune, which still retained the conservative mores of the Peshwas, with strict rules prescribed for Brahmin men, and even stricter rules for women (India had and continues to have a caste system. Brahmins are upper castes with many privileges. Chitpavan Brahmins are a particular sect of Brahmins from Maharashtra. The Peshwas were the ruling dynasty in the Western state of Maharashtra).

Tilak was in favour of universal school education, but like so many nationalists, he believed that advanced education, especially in the sciences, should be reserved for upper-caste men. In 1884, he was a co-founder of The Deccan Education Society, which focused on Indian culture and nationalist ideas. In 1885, the society set up the now famous Fergusson College.

In 1881, Tilak also founded two papers: *The Mahratta*, a weekly English paper, and its Marathi equivalent, *Kesari*. Both papers would be formidable weapons against British rule, but were also used by Tilak and his fellow conservatives as mouthpieces against the education of women.

By 1882, Pandita Ramabai had blazed onto the scene. The fearless Ramabai, as mentioned earlier, did not care a whit for Tilak and his Peshwa codes of conduct. In return, Tilak called her a 'sorceress'[142] who had converted to Christianity.

Ramabai was not afraid to attack the Dharmashastras (Sanskrit texts on law and conduct). She argued that the lack of education for Hindu women was making both them and their children weak and ill. She set up the Arya Mahila Samaj in 1882, an organisation to educate Hindu women. In 1884, a meeting of the Samaj—attended by over a hundred women—called for more girls' schools.

As we saw earlier, the reformer Jotirao Phule had already set up a school for girls of all castes as early as 1848, along with his wife Savitribai Phule. In 1884, M.G. Ranade set up the Huzurpaga girls' school in Pune, along with liberals like

G.K. Gokhale, R.G. Bhandarkar, Vaman Modak and Tilak's own close associate, G.G. Agarkar. All across Maharashtra, women came forward to support the education of girls.

Tilak and his band of conservative Brahmin men continued to object. He believed that education would hinder women from performing their chief duty: being wives and mothers. If an education was to be delivered, it should focus on religious instruction and household skills, he argued. Women were 'incapable of understanding English, history, mathematics and science as it interfered in the natural aspect of a woman's life. So the girls should be taught at the most Sanskrit, sanitation and needlework. Teaching Hindu women to read English would ruin their precious traditional values and would make them immoral and insubordinate,' he wrote in *The Mahratta*.[143]

Insubordinate, of course, was the key word. A highly educated woman from a lower caste was terrifying to Tilak and his band of brothers. Rukhmabai was a threat, a livewire who might encourage Brahmin women to demand education too. Fortunately, Ranade, Agarkar and the other reformers ignored Tilak's suggestions about the curriculum. They believed that women deserved the same education as men. Going a step further, they threw open the school to girls of all castes and religions, who were taught English, mathematics and science from day one. Tilak ranted in the pages of *The Mahratta*, 'Do you seriously hope that our women will do anything in the direction of original literature for centuries to come? I know of very few female names who have added perceptibly to the stock of human knowledge.'[144]

The Huzurpaga Girls High School still survives today. Among its alumni are many early activists, writers, scientists and academics, including anthropologist Irawati Karve, biologist Kamal Ranadive and film director Sai Paranjpe.

But Tilak did not give up attacking women's education in general and Rukhmabai in particular. In 1887, *The Mahratta* was still arguing that women's education should only go far enough to make them good wives and mothers, and not give them airs above their 'station'. 'The object of female education, we need scarcely repeat, is to promote and not impair domestic peace and comfort, and we must confess there are some things in the High School course which, without the attendant compensating features above pointed out (sic), are likely enough to develop in girls vain tastes and make them feel a sense of superiority to their partners. It is not we believe necessary to point out that if this side be allowed to develop in girls, we should not be surprised to find Sarasvatibais and Ratisundaris ready, like the now immortal Rukhmabai, to "wash their hand clean" of Ganpatraos and Madanpals.'[145]

When Rukhmabai wrote her first letter in *The Times of India*, Tilak mocked the unknown writer of the letter, calling her a 'Hindu lady coming to the front in a manly way to take up the cudgels on behalf of the oppressed and downtrodden half of the Hindu community'.[146] When Rukhmabai went on to criticise the laws of Manu, Tilak became alarmed, and *The Mahratta* editorials became more hysterical. He alleged that her letters had been written by someone else trying to overthrow Hindu custom.[147] At the time, of course, Rukhmabai was twenty-one, hardly a schoolgirl. Reflecting age-old Indian attitudes that have scarcely changed, she was clearly old enough to be married but too young to speak for herself.

It is tempting to argue that Tilak was a product of his conservative times. But many of his friends and contemporaries, such as Agarkar and Gokhale, would speak out boldly in favour of women's education. So too would Phule, who argued that women had been kept uneducated by men so they could be controlled, with the aid of Hindu scriptures. 'If a holy woman had written any scripture, then men would not have been able to ignore the due rights of women,' he said.[148]

Tilak's views on women's education would remain unchanged, even as more girls' schools were set up in Maharashtra. As late as 1916, when a women's university was set up by the reformer D.K. Karve, Tilak continued to argue that Hindu women should be educated only to take up household duties.

A Lady Is Not A 'Bullock Or A Cow'

Meanwhile, *Dadaji Bhikaji* v. *Rukhmabai* came up for hearing, its first date set for 17 September 1885 before Justice Robert Pinhey, a progressive British judge due to retire in only three weeks.

Rukhmabai had three lawyers: F.L. Latham, J.D. Inverarity and K.T. Telang. Telang, the only Indian, was an expert on Hindu law and a believer that the shastras could and should adapt to changing times.

Dadaji's counsel relied heavily on the concept of Hindu marriage as a sacrament. 'From the moment of marriage, the Hindu husband is his wife's legal guardian, even though she be an infant, and has an immediate right to require her to live in the same house as him, once she has attained puberty,' he argued.

But these arguments held no ground with Pinhey. His judgement was only a few paragraphs long, but completely unequivocal. In his short, sharp ruling, he said, 'It seems to me that it would be a barbarous, cruel, a revolting thing to do to compel a young lady under those circumstances to go to a man whom she dislikes, in order that he may cohabit with her against her will.'[149]

He noted that the remedy of restitution of conjugal rights 'had no foundation in Indian law and had been transplanted from England into India. I am not obliged to grant the plaintiff the relief which he seeks, and to compel this young lady of twenty-two to go to his house in order that he may consummate the marriage arranged for her during her helpless infancy.'[150]

When Dadaji's counsel pleaded for costs, Pinhey left the court in no doubt about his leanings, chastising the plaintiff for trying to recover an unwilling young lady 'as if she were a bullock or a cow'.[151]

Pinhey's judgement caused great furore amongst Bombay society. It was welcomed by progressives, but bitterly criticised by conservatives who saw it as an attack on Hindu marriages. *The Mahratta* flew into a rage. 'Mr Justice Pinhey has not understood the spirit of the Hindu laws and has sought to introduce the reform by violent means,' said the editorial. It went on to accuse Pinhey of ignoring a vital feature of Hindu marriages: they were arranged by parents or family elders to keep the family together. Thus, they were obliged to place 'certain restraints' upon the social liberty of its individual members. *The Mahratta* argued that the Hindu marriage was a 'contract', and Dadaji had incurred a heavy loss on the marriage; non-restoration of his conjugal rights was a dead loss to him. 'Who is to reimburse him for the pecuniary loss he has suffered,' it asked.[152]

But *The Mahratta* and *Kesari* were not the only newspapers to tear apart Pinhey's judgement. One of the most savage criticisms came from the *Native Opinion*, a Bombay paper edited by Vishwanath Narayan Mandlik, an expert on Hindu law. Like Tilak, Mandlik was not opposed to social reform, but believed political reform should come first.

The prospect of their own dissatisfied wives walking out of their marriages clearly terrified many upper-caste men. 'Millions of Hindu girls married in their infancy may with impunity break the sacred matrimonial bond,' wrote the *Kaiser-i-Hind*, a Gujarati weekly in Bombay, voicing the secret fears of many men, who knew their child brides remained with them only because they had no choice.

But the judgement also had its supporters. *The Times of India* was loud in its defence, even if it was simultaneously condescending to Indian laws. 'With the use of a little firmness and common sense, Mr Justice Pinhey has, in the course of a morning's work, probably done more for the amelioration of the wretched condition of Indian womanhood than has yet been accomplished.'[153] Pinhey had observed that suits for the restitution of conjugal rights were alien to Hindu law, but *The Times of India*, with its colonial mindset, ignored this and went on to denounce Hindu law as barbaric and old-fashioned. Most other Anglo-Indian papers took the same position, failing to recognise that British law was not exactly progressive either.

Meanwhile, Rukhmabai's fiery friend, Behramji Malabari, did not disappoint. Never one to mince words, he described the relationship between Dadaji and Rukhmabai as slave and slave owner. 'Just fancy the little rebel delivered into the hands of Dadaji Bhikaji, his uncles, aunts, sisters and cousins. It makes one's blood curdle only to think of the outrage. If I had a child in that predicament, I would far rather she died before my eyes.'[154]

Marriage Or Jail: A Choice

Pinhey's radical judgement did not hold. The case went on appeal before the appellate bench of the Bombay High Court, before two more British judges, Chief Justice Charles Sargent and Sir Lyttleton Bayley. After lengthy arguments on the duty of a wife, they reversed Pinhey's judgement. Their rationale was that they were obliged to follow Hindu law, which treats the marriage of daughters as a religious duty imposed on parents, and not a contract between consenting parties. In other words, Hindu marriages could not be dissolved.

The case went to Justice Farran for sentencing. By this time, it had dragged on for nearly three years. And then came a shattering blow. Farran ruled that Rukhmabai was to join Dadaji within a month, or face six months' imprisonment.

By then Rukhmabai had made up her mind to take an unprecedented step. She told the court that she would rather be imprisoned than live with Dadaji. Farran, unmoved by this, ruled in favour of Dadaji, arguing that, while Hindu law did not allow for restitution, it did not specifically forbid it either.

Did Rukhmabai understand the implications of her refusal? We must assume she knew the consequences of standing up to power, and was willing to suffer them. Sudhir Chandra explains its significance. 'Extraordinary by any reckoning, Rukhmabai's defiance is even more impressive because it was made before passive resistance had captured either political theory or popular imagination. It further stands out for having been made by a woman when—let alone India where physically as well as mentally respectable women were confined to the zenana—even in the West women's groups were in the early stages of developing a gendered critique of life, and still uncertain about ways of seeking change.'[155]

Backlash From The Conservatives

Rukhmabai's decision outraged Hindu conservatives, and they were quick to respond. Leading the charge, as always, was Tilak in the pages of the *Kesari*. Under his editorship, the *Kesari* ran a series of scathing pieces against Rukhmabai. She was urged to return to her husband

and try to change him, as millions of Indian women have been urged to do. 'She could still accept the court's verdict and by reforming her husband, live happily with him. In this alone consists her true accomplishment,' advised *Kesari*.

Kesari's interest in Rukhmabai was obsessive. It published a stinging burlesque, called 'The Final Scene in the Rukhmabai Farce'. Once again, they compared her unfavourably to the saintly Anandibai Joshi. Anandibai had been greatly praised by *Kesari* and, by extension, Hindu orthodoxy, which found much to admire in her refusal to eat meat or change her clothing despite being overseas. Anandibai was devoted to her husband, as a good Marathi woman should be. And perhaps, more importantly, Anandibai was a Brahmin woman.[156]

Rukhmabai was painted as a fallen woman of dubious morals. 'It is a great sin to equate a dissolute woman with one whose renowned epic would inspire Hindus as long as they maintain their Hindutva,'[157] fumed the *Kesari*. 'Anandibai did not give up even in the minutest bit (sic) her own religion, proper conduct as a woman, or our own customs and conventions. She (Anandibai) realised that otherwise people would call her dharma bhrashta—fallen from religion—that women from her society will not honour her, and as a result she would not be able to secure the good of her sisters and reform them.'[158]

Tilak went further, drawing on his knowledge of Sanskrit and Hindu mythology. 'His editorials not only bristled with barbed phrases, innuendo and sarcasm, but drew upon the rich storehouse of Sanskrit and lore with which he was so familiar, to make his arguments all the more appealing to his tradition-bound public,' explains historian Stanley Wolpert in his 1962 work on Tilak.

Tilak compared Rukhmabai to the eunuch Shikhandi, in the epic Mahabharata, who had been used as a shield for the Pandavas. 'Even as the Pandavas tried to conquer old grandfather Bhishma by putting forward Shikhandi, so also the reformers have the audacity to fire bullets at our ancient religion under the cover of Rukhmabai, with the intention of castrating out eternal religion. We agree with public opinion that government should not interfere with our customs which have been carried on in our society from time immemorial.'[159] Tilak and the nationalists organised a meeting at Hirabaug on 5 June 1887, where speaker after speaker cited authorities on Hindu law from Manu to Yajnavalkya to declare that women needed to be closely guarded, because they were incapable of living independently. The speakers also urged that Rukhmabai and Pandita Ramabai should be punished for 'the same reason that there is punishment for thieves, adulteresses and murderesses'.[160]

Quite what a young woman of twenty-two felt at being thus alienated from her sex, or being attacked so savagely by such a renowned journalist and activist as Tilak, we shall never know. Rukhmabai did not respond to Tilak and maintained a dignified silence. It could not have been easy. It was apparent that the reformers were happy to educate Hindu women, as they had done with Anandibai, but not to have them reap the benefits of education: the ability to make their own decisions. Meanwhile, Rukhmabai began to draw supporters in Britain and the rest of Europe. The famous German professor of Sanskrit, Max Müller, who had already enraged Tilak's band of nationalists by harbouring Pandita Ramabai in his UK home at the time of her conversion to Christianity, wrote to *The Times* in her support. Using his knowledge of Sanskrit to argue that Hindu scriptures did not prescribe child marriage, Müller described the marriage of children 'as an unnatural atrocity' and appealed to the British Parliament to intervene.[161]

In India, the indefatigable Malabari and the rest of Rukhmabai's liberal supporters set up the Rukhmabai Defence Committee—a committee to raise funds and help in her battle.

Caste And Rukhmabai

How much of a role did caste play in the opposition to Rukhmabai? In her letters, she blames the custom of confining marriage to only within a narrow sub-caste for the lack of better marriage prospects. But her biographer and grand-niece Mohini Varde thinks caste did not play a part in her struggle, and instead believes her real battle was against patriarchy and the notion that women should remain at home. Nevertheless, it is hard to conclude that caste did not play a part in her vilification by Tilak and the conservative press. The Bengali monthly *Prachar* wrote that Rukhmabai, a low-caste woman, had got 'the moon in her possession', meaning she was empowered to do anything she wanted. She could cancel her present marriage and wed a saheb (saheb is a term for a British man). *Prachar* went on to sarcastically argue that Hindus were now obliged to take cognisance of the marital affairs of the 'lowest of the low'.[162]

Rukhmabai's rebellion would be alluded to a decade later when, in 1895, Baba Khem Singh, a prominent Sikh leader said, 'Divorce is not allowed nor remarriage except after the death of the husband, and even then among the Hindus of an inferior status. The high caste Hindu looks upon it with contempt and disgust, and anyone practicing it meets with excommunication.' Khem Singh went further. 'Women in this country are never free. Before marriage, they are under guardianship of their parents, after marriage under their husbands, and after their death under their children. So long as their husbands live, they have no right to leave them.'[163]

Kipling And The Imperialists

But not all of Rukhmabai's supporters had pure motives. Amongst her more high-profile backers was the journalist and author Rudyard Kipling. Kipling, and many other British supporters of Rukhmabai, saw her case as a way to justify British rule and the 'white man's burden'.

Kipling wrote an unsigned op-ed in the *Civil and Military Gazette* on 16 April 1887, in which he criticised orthodox Hindu customs, which he said crippled only women and not men. But then he went on to argue that Indians should therefore not be given political representation. He wrote that Hindus could not claim the advantages of Western civilisation while avoiding all its responsibilities with the excuse that they are bound by tradition.

Thus, Rukhmabai's case became, as one historian called it, an 'ideological football'.[164] All she wanted was to be left on her own to study, but she had become a pawn for various powerful forces. On the one hand were the evangelical and colonialist supporters who used her case as a reason to attack Hinduism and argue for imperialism. And on the other were the Hindu conservatives who launched a smear campaign against her, airing her personal life in the papers.

Breaking Free

A few months before Kipling's op-ed, in February 1887, a desperate and weary Rukhmabai wrote a passionate letter to Queen Victoria, a letter which would prove pivotal and win her much support in Britain. It was the fiftieth year of Victoria's ascension—the Jubilee year—and Rukhmabai made a poignant appeal to the queen as a 'mother'. The letter was published in *The Times* and stirred up considerable debate. This letter, unlike her others, was signed.

Once again, her letter was remarkable for the way it savaged social customs that had long gone unchallenged. Rukhmabai was unsparing of the privilege granted Hindu men, who could marry any number of wives, and live with them or not, while women could not remarry or refuse to live with their husbands, even if they were abusive. 'Is it not inhuman that our Hindoo men should have every liberty while women are tied on every hand for ever?' she wrote.

She then went on to appeal to the queen to intervene. 'At such an unusual occasion will the mother listen to an earnest appeal from her millions of Indian daughters and grant them a few simple words of change into the books on Hindoo law?'[165]

But despite her fiery letters in public, in private Rukhmabai had begun to tire of the long fight. In July 1888, she finally arrived at a settlement with Dadaji, according to which she would pay him 2,000 rupees, and he would agree not to compel her to be his wife. She had no stomach for a long court battle.

By now, she was twenty-four. Her contemporaries, Anandibai Joshi and Kadambini Ganguly, with the advantages of upper-caste privilege and supportive husbands, had already forged ahead of her. She had lost years fighting her case in court. It was understandable that now all she wanted was to begin her studies, and no longer be a martyr to the cause of women's education.

Immediately after the settlement, both parties behaved characteristically. Rukhmabai immediately left for the UK to study medicine. Like generations of men before him—and after—Dadaji quickly found himself another wife, this time a more acquiescent one.

How Rukhmabai Brought About The Age Of Consent Act

Back home in India, Rukhmabai's powerful letters propelled a drive for change. Reformists began to pressure the reluctant government to change the laws regarding consent. The tireless Malabari began a signature campaign to raise the age of consent for marriage.

There was massive opposition from Tilak and other Hindu conservatives. Tilak believed in social reform, but he also believed that social reform should come from within Hindu society, bottom up as it were, and not be foisted on them by British lawmakers. He also believed that Swaraj needed to come first, before social reforms, and that reformers needed to change themselves first, before changing others.[166] To be fair, Tilak practised what he preached. He did not marry off his daughters until they were sixteen, which was old for the time. Many other vocal reformers, meanwhile, actually married their daughters off at eight or nine.

But in 1889 came a savage and horrifying case, which made

legislative interference even more urgent and Tilak's arguments redundant. A ten-year-old girl called Phulmoni Dasi died as a result of being raped by her thirty-five-year-old husband, Hari Mohan Maitee. He was found guilty of causing death by a rash and negligent act, but acquitted of rape.

Once again, Tilak rushed in to defend Hindu custom. He argued that the husband could have no knowledge that his act could cause death. As historian Parimala Rao puts it, 'Tilak discussed it in disgusting details. The entire issue of brutality was side-lined by stating that it was not the issue of a brutal husband full of excessive lust.'[167] Tilak made excuses for Maitee in *The Mahratta*. 'On the particular night in question, it is quite probable that his wife happened to be ill or suffering, and in a weak state and the result of his actions was so disastrous to the astonishment and grief of the husband.'[168] But Phulmoni's case shocked the nation so much that Tilak's argument seemed horribly callous.

The cry for government intervention grew ever stronger. Malabari and various other reformers, including Rukhmabai's lawyer Telang, held meetings across the country, urging legislative action. Lawyers, religious experts, writers and other opinion-shapers joined the cause. It was a fraught issue, as conservatives continued to argue that Hindu laws were sacrosanct and could not be touched.

The Age of Consent Act was finally introduced in 1891, raising the age of consent for sexual intercourse for all girls, married or unmarried, from ten to twelve. The reformers had asked for the age to be raised to sixteen, but in the face of opposition from Tilak and his supporters, even raising the limit by two years took tremendous effort.

To the end of his days, Tilak remained fiercely against social reform by legislation. He continued to believe that it was British rule that was the cause of Indian misery, and not early marriage, the treatment of widows, nor the denial of education to girls.[169]

Escape To The London School Of Medicine

Meanwhile, as furious debate raged in India over the right age for women to marry, Rukhmabai was doing what she had fought so hard to do: study. She was helped to travel to Britain by Dr Edith Pechey, one of the Edinburgh Seven, who raised funds for her. Pechey, by then Dr Pechey-Phipson, had gone on to become a senior medical officer at the Madame Cama Hospital in Bombay.

In India, there was considerable demand for native lady doctors to look after women in purdah, but it was still incredibly difficult for Rukhmabai to convince her mother and her grandfather to allow her to go to England. The sad fate of Anandibai, who sacrificed her health for her calling, was often cited. Eventually, her grandfather relented, after laying down three conditions: 'That Rukhmabai should not eat beef, marry an Englishman, or convert to Christianity. Rukhmabai said that she did not find it difficult to fulfil the last two conditions. However, she did not consider eating beef a sin, in contrast to those who went before her.'[170]

Rukhmabai left India on 24 March 1889. She was finally on her way to doing what she had wanted for so long.

The voyage took four long months. London was shrouded in its traditional thick blanket of fog when Rukhmabai arrived. She disembarked in the middle of a real 'pea souper', as such dense fogs are called. The sight was alarming to a woman who had only ever seen bright sunshine. She wrote in her diary, 'It was a foggy day; all street lamps were lit in the middle of the day. How can we call this an afternoon? To me, it was a depressing sight.'[171]

Later, Rukhmabai would be enraptured by snow. 'It was as if everything was covered with thin cotton threads. I innocently enquired of the chambermaid as to what this miracle was. On this instance, she ridiculed me that I could not even recognise snow.'[172]

In London, Rukhmabai was lucky to find lodgings with the McLarens, a progressive and wealthy couple. As a member of parliament, Walter McLaren supported women's education, while his wife Eva was a suffragist, writer and campaigner for women's rights. Between the two of them, they changed Rukhmabai's world, introducing her to writers, progressives and other campaigners of the time. Among others, Rukhmabai met the poet Lord Alfred Tennyson.

The McLarens' lifestyle—filled with discussions, debates, even fights about the rights of women—was to have a huge impact on Rukhmabai. Eva McLaren had her own study where she read, wrote and worked on her own. A 'room of her own'! It was a concept that Rukhmabai had never encountered, but it seemed a thing worth fighting for.[173]

To the end of her days, she would seek out and prefer the company of Europeans, who treated her as an equal and not as a mere woman. She was described thus by an observer in McLarens' circles: 'Small of stature, as all Indian women are, with the peculiar gentle subdued air of the women of Eastern races, she yet is filled with the heroism and the energy of a Viking of old.'

In 1890, Rukhmabai gained admission at the London School of Medicine for Women. At the time, the dean was the venerable Elizabeth Garrett Anderson. In this hothouse of medical talent, Rukhmabai could hardly fail to flourish. The school taught women the same syllabus as was taught to the men. No concession was made for their sex, and they were often taught by male doctors.

No records remain, sadly, of Rukhmabai's student experience, or of her conversations with teachers and peers. But in 1892, Eva McLaren wrote a reassuring letter to Rukhmabai's mother, Jayantibai, 'Words are inadequate to praise your daughter. She has won over our hearts as well as those of our friends... She is studying hard to achieve her objective of becoming a doctor to serve Indian women.'[174] By this time, Rukhmabai had even met the Prince of Wales, who asked her if she enjoyed studying in the UK. Rukhmabai was too overwhelmed to do much beyond reply in the affirmative. Later, she would say simply, 'All of you can easily imagine my feelings of awe.'[175]

Rukhmabai's position in high society and the pampering she received from the British literati caused some annoyance to another woman who had also overcome great odds to get where she was: Cornelia Sorabji, the first Indian woman lawyer. Cornelia and Rukhmabai would go on to have a peculiar relationship.

Cornelia And Rukhmabai

Cornelia Sorabji came from a chequered and fascinating background. Her father, Reverend Sorabji Karsedji, was a Parsi-born Christian missionary, and her mother, Francine Ford, a Parsi woman adopted by a British couple. Cornelia had been the first female graduate of Bombay University, and then, much like Rukhmabai, assisted in her path to the UK by well-wishers. Cornelia was studying law at Somerville College in Oxford as Rukhmabai was being feted by British society.

Cornelia too had wanted to be a doctor but had been discouraged by her mentors and was compelled to choose law instead. In her auto-biography, Cornelia seems resentful and mildly jealous of Rukhmabai's fame, and indeed, despite sharing lodgings for a while, the two did not get along. Rukhmabai visited her at Somerville and Cornelia felt that 'her conversation was one long comparison between us'.[176]

'She most amusingly appeared as the champion of female education in India,' wrote Cornelia to her parents in 1892. 'Did you ever? I suggested that a visit here brought responsibilities, and that we ought to seek usefulness not notoriety and fame. She is quite spoilt and thinks no end of herself.' Later, Cornelia would complain that Rukhmabai had taken to dressing like herself. '[Rukhmabai] has put aside her brown saree and wears red like me now.'[177]

The academic and writer Antoinette Burton seeks to explain Cornelia's strange, unsisterly conduct. 'Given Sorabji's investment in being the only Indian woman doing law, and given Rukhmabai's already "public" reputation in the wake of her trial, distinguishing herself from Rukhmabai through her saris may have seemed the only way to keep her identity, her plans, and her respectability distinct.'[178]

In 1890, the two women went sightseeing together in London. But even here, Rukhmabai could not escape her 'notorious' reputation. Wrote Cornelia, 'She has taken a great fancy to a stuck-up fop from Kolapoor (Kolhapur), the most despicable youth I've ever set eyes on. His name is Mutgatkar. And Miss Bailey told me that he and Rukhmabai wander about the streets together—most disgraceful I call it. That comes of opposing existing laws, and breaking loose from proper restraint.'[179]

The last line was a pointed reference to Rukhmabai's divorce of her husband. Clearly, there were liberal, educated women who were unsympathetic to Rukhmabai. It is difficult to imagine that caste did not play a part in this—the stratospheric rise of a woman from a historically oppressed caste becoming the darling of the British establishment made her many enemies amongst the traditionally more privileged.

Later, Cornelia appeared to have changed her mind, or at least decided to be more diplomatic. In her 1934 memoir, *India Calling*, she wrote that, 'Rukhmabai never read the papers and cared nothing (for the controversy over her case). She had found herself. That was all there was to it—an unusual and fine character, silent and almost stolid. She has served her country with ability and dignity.'[180]

Cornelia also shares an interesting insight as to Rukhmabai's deliberately low profile after she returned to India. 'Throughout her active professional life she remained unemotional and untouched by the hysteria of politics or women's rights.'[181] Perhaps she had had enough of the limelight.

Around this time, Rukhmabai made an unusual and maverick friend: Alice Russell, the then wife of the philosopher Bertrand Russell. Alice Russell was a bluestocking, a highly intellectual woman who preferred reading to conjugal life with Bertrand. Later, Bertrand would divorce her. Before marriage, she belonged to the Peersol Smith family, who had come over from the United States. The Peersol Smiths were Quakers, puritanical, high-minded and believers in simple living.[182] Rukhmabai spent a lot of time with Alice, having in common a distaste for men and marriage. The Quaker lifestyle deeply influenced her, and she decided even then to lead a life of social service. The battle in court had given her a distaste for traditional religion, and she felt a keen interest in changing society.

Pandita Ramabai and other Indian progressives encouraged Rukhmabai to break tradition. Her British education and her exposure to the suffragettes only made her more determined to find her own path: neither British nor Indian, but a happy mixture of the two: an educated woman who would help her own countrywomen as they needed.

Rukhmabai began to raise money with the aim of educating girls in the English language. In 1895, she appealed to the British public to contribute to a society called The Students Literary and Scientific Society of Bombay. The president of the society was M.G. Ranade, and one of its members was Rukhmabai's old ally Behramji Malabari. 'The education of Indian girls over 10 receives but little sympathy even from wealthy native gentlemen,' argued Rukhmabai, adding that the women of India 'know not where else to turn for help.'[183]

It was 7 September 1895. Rukhmabai had finally got her Licentiate of the Royal College of Physicians and was recognised in England's Medical Register. She wrote a letter to the Madame Cama Hospital, expressing her desire to work in India.

By this time, Anandibai had been dead for nearly eight years. In Bengal, Kadambini Ganguly, after graduating from Edinburgh, had been practising for two years. But neither of these women had been completely alone, as Rukhmabai was, or had to face the challenges she did. Held back for longer than the other two, Rukhmabai had a lot to catch up on, and much to demonstrate to her detractors, the traditional Hindus who still tried to shame her for breaking her marriage. It was time to return and do just that: prove herself.

Building A Life In Surat

Rukhmabai returned to India at just the right moment. After she began working at the Madame Cama Hospital, an opportunity presented itself in Surat. The Dufferin Fund was combing India for lady doctors to help Indian patients. Under the scheme, Rukhmabai was offered charge of the Sheth Morarji Vibhukandas Malawi dispensary in Surat, named after a generous donor. Today it is called the Rukhmabai Hospital and her photograph is affixed to a wall.

Rukhmabai was to spend twenty-two years there as its chief medical officer. She lived with dignity and pride and, having broken all the strictures of family, she would set about building her own support group of colleagues and Surat progressives.

Then—as now—Surat was dominated by textile and diamond merchants, who were deeply orthodox. Women lived in quasi-purdah, often not permitted to leave the house. They gave birth at home, in dark and often filthy rooms. But influenced by the progressive movement in Maharashtra, led by Anandibai, Ramabai, Gurubai Karmakar and Rukhmabai, Gujarat was seeing the first faint stirrings towards education and more freedom for women. Rukhmabai became a beacon for the progressive movement.

Her first step was to inspire confidence in women and encourage them to visit her hospital. She was not afraid of taking some very unorthodox steps. At the time, women rarely went to a hospital for delivery, preferring to give birth at home, often in unhygienic conditions. One day, Rukhmabai grabbed a passing pregnant sheep, kept it in the hospital and delivered its lamb.[184] Bizarrely, this helped convince women, and a steady trickle of expectant mothers soon began arriving at the hospital.

In her sparse diary, Rukhmabai wrote about some of the primitive and often unhygienic birth practices of the time. 'I got a call from a Parsi family for the first time… but to attend a whole delivery at their house meant a breaking of the back and one's limbs. There was no chair to sit. All the work had to be done in total darkness on guesses. For forty days, the pregnant women were not allowed to touch wood. Only steel was allowed. My *dai* (midwife) had to sit beside the pregnant woman who had to sleep on the floor. A cot was never offered, though I was given a special concession and offered a one-foot-high stool. We had to sit like that for two nights.'[185]

Rukhmabai went on to talk about other unwise birth rituals.

'There was a strange practice in a lot of Hindu families. The umbilical cord of the baby and the other attached part of the uterus were kept in an earthen pot, which was to be raised (lifted up to the level of the baby) when the baby was breastfed, and preserved until the whole thing dried up. The pregnant woman was made to sleep on dirty grass inside a cow pen. It was only through the grace of God that I was able to deliver babies in such dirty and unhygienic conditions.'[186]

In keeping with her tendency to break rules, Rukhmabai also started a women's group. It seems strange in today's world of women's organisations and satsangs, but in the 1890s, gatherings of women were viewed with deep suspicion. Women were meant to be in the home, taking care of the men, not outside it.

Rukhmabai realised that building the gatherings around religion would give women a socially acceptable reason to attend. Thus, she began organising sessions for women in her house, with the ostensible reason of reading religious books. Gradually, the women began to sew, make chutneys and handicrafts for extra money and read newspapers to find out what was happening in the outside world.

The sisterhood of women grew. One of the women who frequently attended the gatherings was Shivgauri Gajjar. Shivgauri was a seventeen-year-old widow, whose brother encouraged her to attend the meetings to give her a purpose in life. The Gujarat (a state in Western India) of that time was a cruel place for widows, who were shamed and ostracised. Shivgauri idolised Rukhmabai, who showed her that it was possible to make a life for herself outside the limits imposed by society.[187]

Shivgauri would go on to establish the Vanita Vishram home for widows in 1907 with another widow, Bajigauri D. Munshi. The home was open to women of all castes and communities. Despite opposition from conservatives, Vanita Vishram would expand its activities to include women's schools and colleges. Today, the brand has centres across Gujarat and in Mumbai, and has educated thousands of women over the years. And it all began with that small gathering in Surat, ostensibly to sing bhajans, which gave women the courage to step outside their homes.

Rukhmabai continued to be full of surprises. In 1904, Dadaji died. Unexpectedly, Rukhmabai decided to wear the widow's white. Did she want to make one last gesture of reconciliation towards the man she had despised, even though he was dead? Or did she feel widow's garb would help her gain social acceptance? It is hard to say. Either way, she continued to wear white until her death.[188]

Plague And Pestilence

In 1895, only two years into her Surat life, Rukhmabai was faced with a terrifying challenge—the scourge of the century. The plague came to India, and spread like wildfire in Mumbai, Pune and finally, Surat.

The plague was part of the third pandemic, which began in China in 1855. It rapidly spread to port cities across the world, carried by rats on the new steamships. The disease advanced along the tin and opium routes. For the next fifty years, it would appear and disappear, until its eventual end, only in 1959. In that time, it would cause over fifteen million deaths, with the epicentre in India.

The spread of the plague would prompt severe, even savage

measures. Pune was a prime example. The British government invited Ukrainian scientist Dr Walter Haffkine to India to determine the cause of the plague. Working at the J.J. Hospital, Haffkine developed a vaccine for the plague, which he tested on himself. But Haffkine's vaccine was not widely available, or even accepted, and the disease spread faster than the vaccine could be produced.

In 1897, the plague raged through Pune. A Special Plague Committee was formed, under the chairmanship of Walter Charles Rand, an Indian Civil Services officer. Troops were brought in to deal with the emergency. The brutal measures employed included forced entry into private houses and temples, forced stripping of occupants (including women) by British officers in public, evacuation to segregation camps, destroying personal possessions and preventing movement from the city. Rumours spread as fast as the plague, with some believing that the plague was caused by Queen Victoria. The plague was followed by widespread famine.

In this tense atmosphere, the government's measures were seen as imperialist and excessive by many, including Rukhmabai's old foe, Bal Gangadhar Tilak, still as fierce as ever. Tilak wrote editorials in the *Kesari* criticising the British government's measures as invasive and insulting to Hindu women in purdah. Rand was widely despised by Punekars.

A trio of brothers—Damodar Chapekar, Vasudev Chapekar and Balakrishna Chapekar—were enraged by his measures. On 22 June 1897, they shot Rand and his military escort, Lt Ayerst, killing both. The brothers were swiftly arrested, charged with murder and hanged.

The plague, and the measures to deal with it, were thus extremely controversial and emotive. Sadly, for us, Rukhmabai left no written record of how she handled the situation in Surat. But it seems safe to assume that she was forced to take strong and probably difficult measures, as dictated by the government. The government awarded her the Kaiser-i-Hind medal in 1898, which seems to indicate that she did all she could to help victims.

Royalty In Rajkot

In 1917, Rukhmabai left Surat and moved to Rajkot, where she practised at the Rasulkaji Janana Women's Hospital.

She worked with the poor in Rajkot, but also became the darling of several royals. She became the doctor to the rani (queen) of Palitana. The rani lived a luxurious life, eating off Western-style china, with four meals a day served by liveried butlers. Rukhmabai was also introduced to Ranjitsinhji, the royal-turned-cricketer. He lived in a palace with specially constructed tunnels underneath, which hid his stash of treasures: gold cutlery, paintings and flowerpots.

An amusing part of Rukhmabai's life in Rajkot was her difficulty in getting female assistants, despite a burgeoning number of women in medicine.[189] Still, Rukhmabai went through twelve assistants in five years. Her first, an eccentric Parsi woman, would turn up at the hospital 'in her riding outfit, whip in hand, accompanied by her hunting dog', causing consternation amongst the patients. A second lady doctor from the Andamans turned out to be quite idiosyncratic too. Rukhmabai wrote, 'She felt that all her enemies from the Andamans had come chasing her and were now spitting at her. She even used to kick servants in the hospital.'[190]

The third of her assistants was incredibly vain. An exasperated Rukhmabai wrote of how she changed her saris three or four times a day and wore saris with gold and silver borders on Sundays, making her quite unsuited for the gruelling work in the hospital, mostly the delivering of babies.

A fourth assistant quit because she did not want to look at the 'private parts' of women, which made her quite useless for deliveries. A fifth, another Parsi lady, had made various investments in the share market, and spent all her time checking their progress in the newspaper.[191]

Retirement And Legacy

Later, Rukhmabai would retire to Mumbai. She continued to speak out against the purdah system, child marriage and the cloistering of women, and remained a proto-feminist till her death. She published a widely circulated pamphlet called *Purdah: The Need for Abolition*, where she wrote about the need to educate women and give them opportunities.

She would remain wary of marriage until the end of her life, even throwing a dampener on the marriage plans of others. Often, she would 'maintain a studious silence when it came to issues regarding matrimony. Her past had made her a person with a fanatical anti-opinion regarding man-woman relationships,' writes Mohini Varde.[192]

Nevertheless, hers was not a lonely life. She was surrounded by adoring nieces and nephews, and the children of neighbours. She began studying Sanskrit at the age of sixty and became deeply interested in religion and philosophy. The end came on 25 September 1955. She was ninety. Dadaji had been dead for fifty-one years.

Rukhmabai left behind her a remarkable legacy of defiance. It was brave enough for a woman to build her own life in 1884. But for a woman from a lower caste to do it, battling abuse from the entire might of Hindu society, showed fierce determination. Her mentorship of others like her built a whole generation of independent women and served as a model for lady doctors to follow. Upon her death, the British doctor Louisa Martindale, herself a rebel, wrote, 'Unlike some pioneers, Rukhmabai was never aggressive or tactless. On the contrary she was gentle, had great charm and a keen sense of humour. A pioneer of whom her beloved country must be justly proud.'[193]

CHAPTER FIVE

The Fighter

Haimabati Sen

'If the gold medal were to be given to the person who had stood first, it should be Haimabati Sen. But the boys protested... and went on strike. Some said, "Why don't we kill that girl?" It is a great mistake to pamper women.'

Married at nine to a forty-five-year-old. Widowed at twelve. Deserted by her family. Denied an education. Left in grinding poverty. Haimabati Sen's early life was not so different to that of many Indian women. What made her different was that she would—with no encouragement—come up with the idea of becoming a doctor, struggle through a third-rate medical school with no support and somehow endure. Unlike Anandibai and Kadambini, she did not have a supportive husband. Unlike Rukhmabai, she did not have the backing of liberals, support from other lady doctors or help from powerful British women. Unlike them, she did not go to a respected medical school.

She would write an astonishing memoir, unprecedented in its frankness, but would be forgotten by the world, and even her own family. She would find great satisfaction in adopting over three hundred destitute children, and yet spend much of her life struggling to support them. She would fight, but she would mostly fight alone.

We know about Haimabati's life because of her memoir in Bengali, *Because I Am a Woman*—a long-lost treasure that was only discovered and translated very recently. It is a searing, candid and bitter account of the life of a woman in a man's world. Haimabati is amazingly blunt about the double standards for men and women in Hinduism, unlike any woman of her time. She unabashedly calls out her husband for domestic abuse, shames her family for abandoning her and flays Hinduism for its treatment of widows.

Haimabati wrote her memoir in the 1920s. By this time, keeping a journal was fashionable for Brahmo women; she was not a Brahmo, but had adopted many of their socially progressive ways. The memoir, written on hand-ruled notebooks, lay forgotten in a trunk for decades, and was published only eighty years after her death, in 2011. Her relatives did not think it worth publishing, or even reading, and her translator Dr Tapan Raychaudhuri had to persuade them that it was groundbreaking. A photograph of her shows a sturdy, capable-looking woman, broad-shouldered and with a stoic expression. She looks like the stern matriarch of a large family, the kind of woman who could handle anything. And that is exactly who she was.

Chuni Babu: The Girl Who Was A Boy

As in the case of so many Indian girls, it was made clear from the first day of Haimabati's life that she should have been born a boy. Her birth in 1866, in the Khulna district of Bengal, was greeted with tears and disbelief. A dreaded girl! As was the custom, her mother was immediately abused by her grandmother for giving birth to a girl. Worse, her uncle had left an astonishing 5,000 rupees for the first boy in the family, which would now go to someone else.

But her father, Prasanna Kumar Ghosh, a wealthy zamindar (landlord) and an unusual man for the time, rejoiced. He ordered celebrations and lamps to be lit. 'No one must describe my child as a girl. This is the first son born to me.'[194] Haimabati writes how her father treated her with all the respect due to a boy child. 'The servants got together and asked, "What should we call this girl baby?" My father said, "You shall call her Chuni Babu. Or Mr Chuni.'"[195] Indeed, for the first five years of her life, the child Haimabati was dressed like a boy and called Chuni.

Her birthplace, Khulna, is now a bustling port in Bangladesh, in the Ganga-Brahmaputra delta. It is the gateway to the Sunderbans, the mangrove forests, which were alive with man-eating tigers at the time Haimabati was born.

Khulna's most famous resident was probably Khan Jahan, a Sufi saint and nobleman, who came to Bengal after the sacking of Delhi by Taimurlane in 1398. He cleared the forests and made the district suitable for farming. He also built a number of mosques, roads and other buildings, the most famous being the spectacular Sixty Dome Mosque in Bagerhat, now an important tourist destination.

Just over a century after Haimabati's birth, Khulna would become a bloody killing field during the Bangladesh war of 1971. The Pakistan Army would invade the district and massacre the locals before eventually surrendering to Indian forces. Today, a genocide museum stands in Khulna, to remember the atrocities committed by Pakistan on Bangladeshis.

Back in the time of Haimabati, the Bengal famine hit in 1872. Haimabati, only six years old, would go into the storerooms, steal 'large quantities of rice'[196] and give it to the village poor. Later, she would give blankets and mats. Her father supported her, but her mother would beat her every time she caught her. Even when very young, Haimabati felt the intense suffering of the poor. She saw them scramble for rice and boil taro roots to eat. It was to make a lifelong impression on her. After the famine, wrote Haimabati, 'came diseases and epidemics.'[197] Her father brought experienced doctors into the village, stopping the 'quacks' from practising. All this would influence Haimabati.

At the time, there was a superstition that if women were educated, they would become widows. It was a convenient superstition for men, of course, allowing them to keep women under their control. Thus,

Haimabati was not educated, but she eavesdropped on the classes taught to the boys, even though she 'did not know a single letter of the alphabet.'

'I could live like a boy in every other respect, but when it came to education, I was a woman,' she writes wryly.[198]

But one day a sub-inspector visited the school and the young Haimabati answered a question that the boys did not know. The sub-inspector was so impressed by her that he asked her why she was not learning the alphabet. 'Doesn't that lead to widowhood?' asked an innocent Haimabati. 'If that happens, let it,' he replied.[199] The sub-inspector then spoke to her father about educating her. Her father replied that he was willing, but the women in the family were strongly against it. So, they came to an agreement: Haimabati would study in secret.

And so Haimabati's life changed overnight. One of the first books she learned to read was the *Ramayana*. One day she read it before her grandmother and grand-aunts. They were horrified. They immediately complained to her mother.

'See what your hussy of a daughter has done. She is certainly going to be a widow. You are sure to lose caste. She has grown into a masculine woman.'[200] Haimabati ignored them—it was a skill she would learn to cultivate— and went on to win prizes in reading. Each time, she was criticised for her arrogance, and the regular cry 'No one will marry her!' would ring out.

'Buried Alive' In Marriage

By this time, her mother and grandmother had begun attempts to marry her off. A number of bridegrooms rejected her on the basis that she was too educated.

Haimabati's father was on her side. But even he could not withstand the immense social pressure to arrange her marriage. Haimabati belonged to the Kulin Kayastha caste. By custom, they were expected to marry their daughters to higher castes. An unmarried daughter in the house was considered deeply shameful, and a burden on her family. Bridegrooms were expected to be wealthy, accomplished men who could support their brides, which often meant that they were in their forties.

Historian Dr Tapan Raychaudhuri, who also translated Haimabati's autobiography, explains the logic behind the custom of child marriage, a custom adopted even by the reformers. 'If the wife had to accept her husband's family as her own and learn to subject her will to that of others, the relevant process of socialisation had to begin early. Marriage for girls at the age of one to four was not unknown. The brides in the earliest instances of widow remarriage, sponsored by modernising reformers, were aged six to twelve. The cruder arguments in the debate on widow remarriage evoked the age-old belief in the greater lust of women—allegedly eight times as intense as that of men. Child marriage was evidently meant to ensure that this highly disruptive force was contained within the bounds of legitimate conjugal relationship as soon as a young girl became aware of her sexual urge.'[201]

Thus, the inevitable. At nine and a half, Haimabati was married to a forty-five-year-old widower, a deputy magistrate of Jessore, who had already lost two wives and had two daughters around her age. No one saw anything wrong in this massive age gap. Indeed, Haimabati's new husband was considered a catch, because of his wealth and position. Thus began Haimabati's hellish married life. Her helpless father referred to her as being 'buried alive'.

Were the child brides forced to have sex? Says Raychaudhuri, 'The institution of child marriage precluded sex before puberty in pre-modern times, at least in theory. But there is nothing to suggest that sex before puberty did not occur or that it was in fact even frowned upon. A child-bride married at nine or even earlier would often return to her husband's home before she had attained puberty. The data on the sexual side of conjugal relations within the traditional system of marriage as experienced and perceived by women are expectedly limited.'[202]

Haimabati's memoir is thus a singular exception in its brutal frankness about the sex forced on child brides. This was no Anandibai Joshi playing at being a good Indian wife and reluctant to speak ill of her husband. Haimabati would not be shamed, and held nothing back. 'To my knowledge, Haimabati's memoirs are the only account written by a Bengali woman which refers explicitly to matters sexual,'[203] writes Raychaudhuri.

Surreal, terrible days followed. During the day, she and her husband's daughters played with dolls. At night, she would make excuses to avoid her husband's advances.[204]

Haimabati would lie on the bed, silent and stiff as a piece of wood. When she fell asleep, someone would remove her clothes. She would wake up and wrap herself in a blanket.[205] Haimabati's husband continued to bring prostitutes home at night as she cowered in a corner. One night, the woman her husband brought home scolded him for having sex in front of his sheltered young child bride. 'How else will she learn?' responded the unrepentant husband.[206]

The young Haimabati was so traumatised that she began to faint and have strange dreams. She was hastily sent to her parents' house to recover. Her account of this stay makes tragic reading. She continued to faint in her father's house, and her mother began to believe that she was possessed by a spirit. An exorcist was summoned who beat her. Her furious father beat him up and sent him packing.

But her father was helpless and vented his deep frustration at having to send her back to her husband. 'Spirit possession indeed! Like hell! Because of your pestering, I threw her into deep water with her hands and feet tied before she had grown up. Now if she dies, let her. I shall not do anything about it. Let her die. She will suffer a lot more if she survives.'[207] Haimabati's father's rant is a never-before-recorded picture of the manner in which child marriage trapped and imprisoned entire families, even progressive ones.

A Child, A Widow, An Outcaste

Once again, Haimabati was summoned back to the side of her husband, even more terrified. Her husband tried to make overtures to her, but a traumatised Haimabati began to shout loudly when asked to sit by him, despite being chastised by her family.

Only a day or so later, Haimabati's life would be turned upside down. Her husband got a fever. It turned out to be pneumonia. For three weeks, they nursed him. Her husband finally began to feel sorry for her. 'You have no idea what disaster I have caused you. You are a mere child. Who will look after you?'[208]

But it was too late for him to make amends. A few days later he was dead, and Haimabati was that most inauspicious and pitiable of things: a child widow.

Her deep, overwhelming rage at this turn of events is magnificent. She does not mince words. 'No one gave a thought as to what would happen to the life of this girl? There was no one to say a word of pity to me. Some days I ate, others I just lay in a corner. My parents had fulfilled their duty towards me. No one was responsible for this child widow. If I needed a single pice, I would have to beg it from others. What about my husband? He had taken a third wife and cut a child's throat. What provision had he made?'[209]

A furious Haimabati went on to flay Hindu customs. 'Shame on you, Hindu society. A girl of ten will have to pay for the marriage of an old man of fifty. In no other country does one find such conduct; such oppression of women is possible only in India.'[210]

Haimabati was, of course, not alone in enduring early widowhood. With most Kulin Kayastha brides being thirty years younger than their husbands, a new child bride could expect in most cases to soon be a child widow. A widow would be shunned and mistreated at best, and raped or abused at worst. They would have their heads shorn, wear only white for the rest of their life and live in crushing poverty. Many would be denied claims to their husband's properties and turn to prostitution to survive. In 1853, it was estimated that Calcutta had a population of 12,718 prostitutes, many of them child widows.[211]

If only Haimabati had known, a few reformers in the Hindu society she so despised were rebelling against the treatment of widows. A hundred kilometres away, in Calcutta, change was coming, though at a glacial pace. People had begun to discuss the hard questions that Haimabati had raised.

Vidyasagar And The Winds Of Change

Behind the movement was one of the most interesting and brave of Indian reformers: the scholar Ishwar Chandra Vidyasagar. Born Ishwar Chandra Bandyopadhyay in a poor family, Vidyasagar had been deeply affected by the marriage of one of his tutors, a forty-something man, to a girl of eight. He urged the tutor to reconsider, but he refused. Within a year, the tutor was dead, and his girl bride widowed. Vidyasagar himself was married at age fourteen to a girl of ten, and his protests were ignored by his family.

A stern-faced man with a massive, egg-shaped forehead, Vidyasagar would do more than any other to encourage widow remarriage. A professor of Sanskrit and the principal of the Sanskrit College in Calcutta, he realised that only Hindu texts would persuade people to change their minds. So he spent hours unearthing obscure shlokas (Sanskrit verses) that would support his position. In 1854, he wrote an article in a progressive journal called *Tattvabodhini Patrika*, in which he quoted the shloka 'Parashar Dharma Samhita', said to be written by the sage Parashar. The shloka stated:

The Fighter

Gate Mrite
Pravajite pleevache patit patau
Panchasvapatsu narinam patiranyo bidhiyate

Translated, it means, 'Women are at liberty to marry again, if their husband is not heard of, dies, retires from the world, proves to be impotent, or be an outcast.'[212]

People were shocked, but Vidyasagar was encouraged by men who had gone before. Raja Ram Mohan Roy, the great reformer and one of the founders of the Brahmo Samaj, had already shaken up Bengali society with his immensely unpopular views.

Like Vidyasagar, Roy had been deeply affected by an incident in his childhood. In 1811, Roy's much-loved sister-in-law was burnt on the pyre of her dead husband. Roy would grow up to campaign against sati (a practice by which Hindu widows self-immolated themselves on a pyre, sometimes voluntarily but often coerced by families), and actively work for the education of women and the banning of child marriage. In 1829, despite strong opposition from Bengali orthodoxy, he would succeed in paving the way for Governor General William Bentinck's Bengal Sati Regulation, banning sati throughout India.

Vidyasagar thus had a precedent for trying to enforce an unpopular law. He began to gather signatures for a petition to change the laws relating to widow remarriage. Such was the opposition to the idea that he could gather only 1,000 signatures. Against the proposition were 30,000 signatures.

One of the main opponents of widow remarriage was Radhakanta Deb, a social conservative, who was also a long-standing enemy of Raja Ram Mohan Roy. In 1829, Deb, along with other conservatives, had started the Dharma Sabha to protest the abolition of sati and counter other social reform movements. They specifically protested the abolition of sati because they did not believe in interference in Hindu affairs. Ironically, Deb was in favour of educating girls. But he also believed that the wave of social reform led by Raja Ram Mohan Roy, and later Vidyasagar, would destroy and weaken the Hindu way of life. Instead, he argued that reform should come from within. Deb's preference for 'reform from inside' would be a popular stance with future Hindu conservatives like Bal Gangadhar Tilak.

Eventually, the British government decided that the 'enlightened minority' would prevail. The Widow Remarriage Act was passed in 1856, giving Hindu widows the right to remarry. But as Vidyasagar was to find out, enacting a law was one thing. Getting society to accept the idea of widows remarrying, or even getting them to treat widows humanely, was another. The law remained effective only on paper.

Vidyasagar continued to put out pamphlets arguing his case. One such was an 1885 pamphlet, titled, *Whether the Practice of Widow-marriage among Hindus Should or Should Not Prevail*. It lamented, 'How many hundreds of widows, unable to observe the austerities of a Brahmacharya life [a lifestyle which involves renunciation of marriage and sex, usually prescribed for widows and monks], betake themselves to prostitution and foeticide and thus bring disgrace upon the families of their fathers, mothers and husbands. If widow-marriage be allowed, it will remove the insupportable torments of life-long widowhood, diminish the crimes of prostitution and infanticide and secure all families from disgrace and infamy. As long as this salutary practice will be deferred so long will the crimes of prostitution, adultery, incest and foeticide flow on in an ever increasing current… so long will a widow's agony blaze on in fiercer flames…'[213]

It is true that Vidyasagar was partly motivated by a prudish Victorian mentality. He was shocked by the idea that widows might be sexually independent, and by the profusion of child widows turning to prostitution. He also did not consider that widows had limited property rights, and thus did not make this aspect a part of his fight. Still, he was brave enough to do what no one else was doing at the time.

Abandonment And Disgrace

In her little village of Khulna, Haimabati remained unaware of these events. Her memoir contains no mention of Vidyasagar or his reforms. When she returned to her parents' home after her husband's death, she was greeted with abuse from her mother and other relatives. 'They had no sympathy for me; their lamentations were for that old drunkard and whore-monger who had been their son-in-law for only a few days,' she writes in her memoir.[214] She was criticised incessantly for having got an education, for jumping out of the bridal bed and for having been widowed after only a year.

Haimabati began to return to her books, her one comfort. Once again, she was criticised for studying by the ladies. 'What, you are studying again? This is how you brought ruin on yourself and now you are studying again?' But the determined Haimabati snapped back. 'This time I became Kali, the terrible goddess,' she writes. With incredible courage, she replied, 'I cannot be widowed again. What has to happen has happened. You can do whatever you please—kill me or thrash me—but this is what I am going to do.'[215]

The women complained to Haimabati's father, but as always, he was on her side and she was left alone to study. But then came disaster. In the space of less than a year, Haimabati's beloved father, her mother-in-law and her mother all died. Her mother left behind an eighteen-month-old sister for her to take care of. Haimabati's feckless and greedy brother and uncle grabbed the money left behind by her father. Her husband's elder brother rejected her claim to her husband's money, even as she begged for only 10 rupees a month.

Now began Haimabati's long struggle to support herself, as relative after relative conspired to cheat her. This was true penury. She ran from one to the other, trying to get her due, and was rejected at every turn. Her account of this time makes for hard reading. She was still only about twelve years old, but she already knew the price of every handful of rice, every glass of milk, because of how little money she had.

Eventually, Haimabati was driven to take the extreme step: to do what widows were expected and often forced to do. Desperate and alone, she gave up her claim to her husband's and father's estate, and went to Benaras.

Benaras: City Of Widows

Benaras in the 1880s. What would Haimabati have seen? Her account of this time is very practical, only mentioning the process of trying to extract money from her family and the humiliations heaped upon her. She says nothing about the city of Benaras. But if Haimabati had had the time or the energy to look around, there would have been much for her to marvel at.

The British writer and art historian E.B. Havell, Haimabati's contemporary, wrote memorably about the Benaras of the time in his book, *Benares, the Sacred City: Sketches of Hindu Life and Religion*:

> At Manikarnika, we reach the central point of the ghats: the very pivot of the religious life of Benares. There is perhaps no more extraordinary sight in this world than the ghat presents any morning in the month of Karthik, or at any great Hindu festival. Shrines innumerable, cut in the stone piers and terraces which project into the stream; temples at the water's edge, half sunk in the stream, temples on the ghat steps, the five-spired temples of Durga crowning the high ridge above. The burning ghat, black with the smoke of funeral pyres; corpses laid out by the river on their rough biers of bamboo. A few yards away, the women's bathing ghat, glowing like a flower garden with the colours of their saris. Pilgrims from every corner of India, carrying their bundles with them, are arriving at the sacred well, brought there by the *Gangaputras* to begin their round of devotions,

which is often preceded by clamorous disputes for the fees
their spiritual preceptors demand.[216]

In Benaras, Haimabati approached a distant relative, now that her own relatives had disowned her. Pulin Babu was her cousin's husband, and he assured her that he would give her 20 rupees every month.

Haimabati had thought that she would be accepted in Benaras, the city of widows. But she soon learnt how widows were really viewed, under the sanctimonious veneer of piety and duty. Her cousin immediately objected to her stay. 'You are a widow but you are also young and beautiful. What will people say if you stay with us? Who can guarantee there will be no liaison between the two of you? Such liaisons are very common in Benaras.'[217]

A weeping Haimabati did what she would do many times in her life: throw herself on the mercy of strangers. In her experience, they would often be kinder to her than her own family. She took refuge in the home of the wife of the priest at her cousin's home, who found her lodgings with a respectable family. By this time, Haimabati was living hand to mouth. But she would not ask for help.

'I would buy a *pice* worth of wood and cook three handfuls of rice with salt. That was all I ate. I did not eat anything at night. If anyone asked me, I would say, "As a widow I cook but once a day." When people heard this they concluded I ate nothing but rice in accordance with the requirements of a spiritual life. I decided there was no point in letting people know my actual situation. Why should I announce my poverty when no one would help me?'[218]

Haimabati managed to land a teaching job at a girls' school. She remained there for eight months, earning a salary of 10 rupees per month. She found earning her own money deeply satisfying. 'Great was my happiness the day I received my first pay from the school. I wept for joy and handed the money to my aunt. She bought me some snacks in the evening and I ate with a deep sense of contentment.'[219] To stand on her own feet, even on a meagre salary, was no small thing for Haimabati.

But her constant yearning to learn more could not be quelled. She began to dream of educating herself further in the city of dreams: Calcutta. In this, Haimabati was remarkably unusual for her time. Women, especially child widows in the 1880s, did not pursue education. But her life would be marked by a desperate quest to learn more, know more, do more and see more: experience the world in all its glory and pain. It would be both her curse and her redemption. 'Once again I was courting misery,' she writes, uncertainly. 'Who knew what this desire for higher education would bring?'[220]

Haimabati was also propelled to leave Benaras by the ugly reality of life in the town, where young widows were often easy targets for predatory men. Twice, she narrowly escaped being harassed by local goons. Education and earning her own money seemed the only escape.

Remarriage To A 'Saint'

Haimabati's memoir is vague about dates, but by now she was about twenty-two or twenty-three. Now began a strange phase of her life. Haimabati was naturally drawn to the Brahmo Samaj, which believed in the education and remarriage of widows. As historian and author Geraldine Forbes explains, 'Deprived of help from her own and her husband's family, Hem (Haimabati) turned to strangers and made them her kin. In a pattern she would follow throughout her life, Hem called friends and acquaintances "Mother", "Father", "Uncle", "Aunt", "Brother", "Son" or "Daughter".'[221] Most of these people that she would turn to were stalwarts of the Brahmo Samaj.

Haimabati travelled to Calcutta with two letters of introduction to leading members of the Brahmo Samaj, who had helped widows in the past. But once again she was plagued by bad luck. Both the men turned out to be travelling to the UK. Not knowing where to go, Haimabati went with another 'uncle', a friend of a friend. She ended up in East Bengal, in Dhaka, cooking and helping various families with their children. She calls these chapters 'Wanderings in East Bengal', and that they certainly were. The restless Haimabati moved from house to house, weathering suspicion and abuse, ill treatment and poverty.

By this time, Haimabati had also begun to be interested in learning medicine. She does not mention Kadambini Ganguly in her memoir, but by the late 1880s, Calcutta Medical College had opened its doors to women. Across the country, in Bombay, Cornelia Sorabji had created history by being the first woman to graduate from Bombay University. By 1888, Chandramukhi Bose, one of the first two women graduates of the British Empire along with Kadambini Ganguly, had even become the first woman principal of Bethune College. The Brahmos were leading the way in education for women—another reason for Haimabati to cling to them.

But who would pay for this education? Haimabati had begun to realise a cold hard truth: the only way for her to access education would be to marry again. The Brahmos she had thrown her lot in with were modern enough to believe in the education of women. But they were also old-fashioned enough to believe that widows should be remarried, with a man to watch over them.

Haimabati began to come around to the idea. It was 1889 and she was twenty-three. A man named Kunja Behari Sen, a Brahmo missionary of around the same age, had proposed marriage. She was tired of her uncertain, restless life, and probably a little lonely. 'How long can I go on moving from one home to the other? I shall feel secure if I depend on one person,'[222] Haimabati muses in her memoir.

Unfortunately for Haimabati, Kunja Behari was not that person. For their first meeting, he wore saffron clothes, which should have indicated what way his priorities lay. Haimabati saw it as a sign that he was unworldly and pure of heart. She was later to realise that it was a sign of his utter fecklessness and disinterest in family life. For most of their married life, they would live entirely on Haimabati's earnings. Kunja Behari would come and go, mostly go. He would spend a great deal of time on spiritual retreats in the Himalayas, while the practical Haimabati would keep the house going on her salary.

Right after they were married, Kunja Behari informed Haimabati that he had taken a vow of celibacy for six months. He left her in a hostel, while he spent six months helping famine victims. Initially, Haimabati found Kunja Behari's do-gooder ways endearing. 'I felt a deep respect for my husband,' writes Haimabati. 'People worry about their own happiness, how many were as self-sacrificing as he was?'[223]

But the novelty of being married to a saint soon wore off. Kunja Behari lost his job with the Brahmo Samaj, and once again, Haimabati was poor and living on the charity of strangers. By this time, she was also pregnant.

The baby came when the couple was unprepared, and it was born dead. They wept over its tiny body, but they had no time to grieve. Haimabati had a bad case of fever: most likely puerperal fever. It was during this terrible situation, broken and on the verge of death, that she met a man who had a deep impact on her.

The man who would save Haimabati's life, and kindle her interest in social service, was Dr Sundari Mohan Das. Das was well known in the Brahmo movement for his dedication towards maternity services, and his championing of women's health. He would write a book, whimsically titled *Briddha Dhatri Rojnamcha* (Diary of an Old Midwife). Years later, he founded Calcutta National Medical College.

His wife, Hemangini, was a midwife. Together, they saved Haimabati's life, refusing to take any money from her. Haimabati came to rely on Das for help whenever her husband went on his travels. The couple would greatly influence Haimabati's path. As she lay recovering after the difficult birth, her fierce—and sometimes unwise—commitment to social service was born.

The Campbell Medical School: Creating Lady Doctors

After the loss of their baby, the hard business of living began again Kunja Behari wanted to work with the Brahmo Samaj for no pay but his meals. 'I shall not do anything but serve god,' he said. Haimabati was weary of depending on charity or turning to strangers again. This time, she would make her own way.

She decided to join the Campbell Medical School to become a hospital assistant. Kunja Behari, with no income, could hardly object. Indeed, he did not care, being totally absorbed in his spiritual pursuits.

The Campbell Medical School had been through several avatars. It was located in Sealdah, which was at that time on the outskirts of Calcutta and thinly inhabited. How did Sealdah get its name? It is uncertain, but historian Thankapan Nair says the name was derived from the words 'sial', for jackal, and 'dihi', meaning village.[224]

The medical school was founded as the Sealdah Medical Hospital in 1873, but was more commonly called the 'paupers' hospital' because it provided shelter to the truly poor and destitute of Calcutta, including smallpox victims. Hence its remote location. In 1884, it was renamed the Campbell Medical School. Then, after 1950, it was renamed the Nil Ratan Sircar Medical College, after a famous alumnus, an education-ist. Indeed, the college had many notable male graduates, who would go on to make major scientific discoveries. In 1912, Dr Kedarnath Das would invent the Bengal forceps, an instrument for delivering babies in Bengali women, who generally had smaller pelvic sizes than Western women. In 1922, Dr Upendranath Brahmachari discovered the antibiotic urea stibamine, used to treat kala-azar.

But these tales of heady achievements were those of the men. It was a completely different experience for the women. Campbell Medical College summed up all the challenges of teaching and training 'lady doctors'. Indeed, the women it trained were not really doctors in the conventional sense. There was all the difference in the world between the highly educated Kadambini Ganguly—the genteel darling of the

Brahmos—and the poorly educated, scrappy loner Haimabati. In 1885, as we know, the Dufferin Fund was set up to provide medical care for Indian women. Initially, it recruited British women and the much-respected graduates of Calcutta Medical College, like Kadambini. But, as historian Geraldine Forbes points out, the Dufferin Fund soon began to run into trouble, not dissimilar to the problems faced by rural hospitals today. It could not find doctors willing to work in rural districts. 'Neither British women doctors nor graduates of the Calcutta Medical College wanted to work where they were most needed—in the districts—or for the low wages proposed. These women stayed in the cities where they worked in large urban hospitals or engaged in private practice. In either case they could easily command salaries ten times those offered by district boards.'[225]

The Dufferin Fund needed to find willing lady doctors for the districts, who would work for a pittance in the most gruelling conditions. The Brahmo Samaj came up with the idea of training less educated women as hospital assistants, who were awarded the VLMS, the Vernacular Licentiate in Medicine and Surgery, a much less exacting qualification than the BAs women like Kadambini Ganguly and Abala Das had. However, British officials doubted there would be suitable applicants. They argued that religion, caste and the purdah system would mean that no Indian woman would sign up.

Even with the Brahmo campaign to get more women into education, there were not enough educated Bengali women. Because of this, standards had to be lowered. There was huge opposition from the medical profession, both from British as well as Indian doctors. The Indian Medical Service was concerned that the entrance examination for women was so dumbed down that they would be totally unfit to practice medicine.[226] They were also worried that 'half-educated' women would bring Western medicine and practices into disrepute.

Eventually, Campbell's superintendent Colin Mackenzie was persuaded to admit women in 1888, five years after the Calcutta

Medical College opened its doors. There were fifteen women in the first batch, mostly Christians and Europeans, with the odd Brahmo woman.

The fears expressed by doctors about the lowering of standards were not entirely unfounded. The exam Haimabati had to pass was ridiculously easy. It had to be, because most women of the time received no science education whatsoever. The majority did not even have a basic education. She had to explain a Bengali book, take dictation and do some very basic arithmetic. While the women enrolled at Calcutta Medical College followed a scientific curriculum, the hospital assistant course introduced only elementary chemistry and physiology.

Even with such an easy course, many dropped out because of circumstances: the women faced huge difficulties trying to balance family and education. Nearly all of them were already married or widowed and had families to take care of. Many were the sole breadwinners. Despite this, the programme proved effective. Between 1891 and 1905, fifty Bengali women graduated from Campbell. According to the 1904 report of the Bengal branch of the Dufferin Fund, thirty-eight of its female hospitals and dispensaries were headed by women who had earned the VLMS degree, and most had graduated from Campbell.

While the Campbell graduates were able to work at new hospitals and dispensaries, they were not allowed to practice on their own. At work, they were supervised by civil surgeons. These women often worked with traditional practitioners of medicine, the dais and the Ayurvedic doctors, and confined themselves to pain relief and childbirth. Gradually, the medical establishment began to accept them, despite their initial outrage.

However, the fact remains that the Campbell lady graduates were often raw and poorly trained in other aspects of medicine. The male doctors treated men with Western medicine and scientific methods. The women were treated by often half-trained 'lady doctors'.

As Forbes baldly puts it, 'They (the medical establishment) toler- ated half-trained women doctors, I believe, because they essentialised both women and science, concluding that pure science was not meant for women. In the end they decided women's bodies could be mended with a few basic concepts and techniques from Western medicine, while science and modernity could be reserved for the men.'[227]

Lady Doctors As Pawns

Half-baked though their training may have been, Haimabati put everything into her studies. Seventeen ladies sat the entrance examina- tion, and Haimabati came second. A woman called Swarnalata Mitra came first, and Idinessa Bibi came third. Most of their teachers were British and difficult to understand for the poorly educated girls. She wrote, 'Our classes in anatomy, materia medica, and surgery began. We had to go in the morning and take lessons in dispensing medicine, but we hardly learned anything because we could not understand what Mr Gibbons said or did.'[228] The three top-ranked women—Swarnalata, Haimabati and Idinessa—were resourceful. They paid a dispenser 3 rupees a month to help them learn dispensing and studied together. The teachers, writes Haimabati, were kind to her. Soon Haimabati was urged to apply for a scholarship.

She did so, and won a scholarship that came to about 7 rupees per month. 'I brought it home and handed it over to my husband, and he spent it the way he considered best.'[229] This was a pattern that would continue throughout their married life. Haimabati would earn the money, and then be forced to hand it over to Kunja Behari. For all her independent ways, she could not escape the shackles of marriage. She had to cook for the feckless Kunja Behari, look after the house and—as always with her—also ended up looking after the children of a neighbour who was a widower. This often meant she stayed up working till half past two.

Haimabati writes an amusing account of her dissection class.

'What we saw there was enough to make us and our ancestors up to the fourteenth degree throw up everything we had ever eaten. The upper half of a male body lay on the table with his entrails hanging out. We burst into tears out of fear and revulsion.'[230]

To the credit of the teachers, there was no special treatment for the girls. 'Jogendra Babu put a knife in my hand, held it, made me remove the skin from the corpse,' wrote Haimabati. 'He said, "Imagine this is an animal. You have to do this for your studies. There is no room for shyness, revulsion or compassion. Think only of your studies. There is no reason to feel scared."'[231]

By this time, Haimabati was pregnant again. She found it immensely difficult to juggle her home and her studies. She was constantly ill and out of breath. For her final examination, Haimabati was evaluated by a British doctor, Dr Bancot, who had once stated that he did not care for female students. By the end of the examination, he had changed his mind and was lavish with his praise.

Haimabati stood first in the examination, with a boy called Gopalchandra Datta half a mark behind. But then hell broke loose. The gold medal was to go to Haimabati, but the boys protested. 'The gold medal prize began long before there were girl students, if it is given to a girl, the boys will go on strike,'[232] they argued. When Mr Gibbons, the superintendent of the college, stood firm, the boys went on strike. 'Some said, "Why don't we kill that girl? That would be the end of the matter. It is a great mistake to pamper women."'[233] For a week, the boys formed pickets, overturned benches and threw bricks and stones at the women students. Gibbons wanted to call the police, but the teachers were against it.

Today, male doctors throwing stones at their female counterparts may seem completely incredible, but across the world, male students were afraid of the competition from female students, who were often more intelligent and worked much harder. Only about twenty years earlier, the Edinburgh Seven had been abused and threatened by the male students at their university. By the time Haimabati entered college, women were grudgingly accepted, but certainly not allowed to be better than the men.

Haimabati was summoned by the lieutenant governor of Bengal, in what can only have been a terrifying experience. She took along her newborn baby, Dhrubajyoti. They tried to strike a bargain with her. 'What do you want if we give the gold medal to one of the boys?' Ever practical, Haimabati could see no use for a gold medal if it made her unpopular amongst her peers and the target of threats from the boys. What she really needed was money for her baby. 'Sir, I am the wife of a poor missionary and have no use for a gold medal. If you want to be kind to me, allow me to continue my studies,' she said.[234]

Haimabati was allowed to continue her studies and her scholarship amount increased to 30 rupees per month as a sop, with the Campbell bus directed to take her to college and back. She was given a silver medal for, as she dryly writes, 'standing first in class'.[235] The male students were appeased.

Haimabati's memories of this time are a vivid portrayal of the problems of a working woman. She took Dhrubajyoti to college and paid a woman to look after him, but it was not easy. Then, with perfect timing, the restless Kunja Behari decided to go to the hills again, for spiritual contemplation. Kunja Behari would periodically set out on trips like this every time the demands of married life and fatherhood got too much for him. He was happy to live off Haimabati's earnings, and contributed very little to the household.

Haimabati scraped along on the scholarship amount she got, but it was paid only every three months. While Kunja Behari was away, she found it impossible to pay her rent and her food. Often, she ate nothing, saving her money for the child. She had only one sari to wear and was forced to beg her neighbours for another. Once again, she was helped by members of the Brahmo Samaj—her extended family.

When her husband returned, Haimabati was angry, and her

memoir reflects this. But she could say nothing to him, trapped as she was in the role of a good Hindu wife. 'My husband came home and immediately began to ride his high horse. [He said] Women are but thorns on the way of life, hindrances to spiritual quest,' she complained. An elderly lady of the samaj told him off. 'If you have decided to spend your life in spiritual pursuits, why did you marry?'[236] As usual, the indifferent Kunja Behari had no answer. But Haimabati had ceased to expect one.

Finding A Job: Bottom Of The Heap

Haimabati passed her final examinations, once again ranking first. Lord Elgin, the viceroy of India, and his wife were present at her graduation. She was awarded a VLMS, a Vernacular Licentiate in Medicine and Surgery.

Now came the next hurdle: finding a job. The hierarchy for doctors was clear: first came the British male doctors, then the Indian male doctors, then the elite lady doctors who had passed out of the Calcutta or Madras medical colleges or had been trained in British colleges. As a hospital assistant, Haimabati was at the bottom of the pecking order. The best she could hope for was to work in a district hospital or dispensary at much lower pay.

Nevertheless, Haimabati was offered a job at the then incredible salary of 200 rupees per month. But Kunja Behari stood in her way— he refused to give up his 'work' at the Brahmo Samaj. By this time, the couple were in debt. Haimabati's son was constantly ill and needed expensive medicines. She tried to set up her own private practice, but people preferred to go to male doctors who had their own midwives.

Haimabati's memoir is singular in its frank account of how lady doctors were often cheated out of their fees. She writes of an incident where a Dr Dayal Shome took her along for a birth by a 'petite European lady', which was also attended by European doctors. The European doctors were keen on a caesarean, but Dr Shome insisted on waiting. The mother groaned in pain, as Haimabati looked on in sympathy. 'Ah, for the mother's heart.' After more than twenty-four hours in labour, Haimabati and the midwife present delivered a healthy child. Haimabati was paid only 50 rupees, while the midwife got 150 rupees and Dr Shome made a whopping 1,000 rupees. Kunja Behari was pleased with the money—50 rupees in a single day—but even though it was more than she had ever made in her life, Haimabati felt she had been short-changed. She was deeply hurt that she had been paid less than the unqualified midwife after all her years of hard work. Haimabati was a woman who knew her worth, and was determined to get what she was due. 'This was the situation of women doctors and midwives in Calcutta. They could get cases [only] with the help of a doctor, and when it came to fees, the doctor took the lion's share,' she complained.[237]

For a woman of her time, with years of poverty behind her, Haimabati was unusual in wanting equal pay with men. 'Lady doctors,' she writes, 'were pawns in the hands of male doctors. When I thought of these things, I lamented the fact that we were born as women.'[238]

As so often in Haimabati's life, the Brahmo Samaj came to her rescue. She had taken her ailing son to see Debendranath Tagore, a leading member of the Samaj. Tagore lived in Chinsurah, a small town about 35 km from Calcutta, on the banks of the Ganga. Haimabati loved it at first sight. When Tagore heard of Haimabati's search for a job, he spoke with other members of the Brahmos about setting up a women's hospital in Chinsurah, under the auspices of the Dufferin Fund. The Hughli Lady Dufferin Hospital was set up, with fifty beds, and Haimabati was appointed. Her salary was 50 rupees per month, much less than what she could have got elsewhere, but still a substantial sum for that time.

Working Life At The Lady Dufferin Hospital

Chinsurah was where Haimabati would spend the rest of her working life. Between the 17th and 19th centuries, it was a trading post for the

Dutch East India Company, who set it up to trade in spices, cotton and indigo. It was called 'The Europe on the Ganges' because it attracted so many Europeans. There still survives a Dutch cemetery, with about forty-five graves. The town is dotted with Indo-Dutch architecture, and was once dominated by a massive fort, called Gustavus. Little of it remains. Now the most well-known attraction is the tomb of Susannah Anna Maria, a Dutch lady who is supposed to have had seven husbands, and was the inspiration for Ruskin Bond's novel *Susanna's Seven Husbands*.

By the time Haimabati arrived, the town had also become known for its nationalist connections. The poet Bankim Chandra Chatterjee studied in the nearby Hooghly Collegiate School, and composed his much-loved anthem, *Vande Mataram*, while living in the town.

Haimabati, ever the maverick, did not shy away from describing her difficult work conditions in her memoir. Not for her the veiled references employed by other women. Today we think of lady doctors as respected professionals, hovering in spotless white coats. Back then, things were very different. Sexual harassment was common for these early professionals making their way into the world of men. Haimabati was constantly harassed by the assistant surgeon of the hospital, one Badrinath Mukherjee. 'The assistant surgeon would talk rubbish. He began with a lesson on diseases, and moved to the topic of shameful [venereal] diseases. One day I protested. "You must not talk of these things to me." He reported this to the boss in a twisted form. The boss asked, "Why are you annoyed when he tries to instruct you?" I only said, "Sir, please ask him not to bring up obscene cases,"' wrote Haimabati.[239]

The Hughli Lady Dufferin Hospital accepted all patients, including the very poor. This meant that more well-to-do women would not visit the hospital, so lady doctors would often visit them in their homes. In the initial years, Haimabati treated about 230 patients a year in the hospital, fifteen times that number in an external clinic, and about 150 patients in their homes. Ten years later, she was treating 400 patients in the hospital, about 6,000 in the clinics, and 270 in their homes. She mentions that she was earning 300 to 400 rupees per month, an immense sum at the time, but all of it was handed over to her husband, who controlled her earnings with a tight fist. She could not spend 'even a *pice*' without asking him for permission.[240]

Haimabati also had to be constantly vigilant of attempts to smear her reputation and the resentment of many hospital staff. Her memoir speaks of Machiavellian plots by hospital clerks, dressers and compounders. Once, for instance, she was asked to attend a patient in another town, the younger brother of a doctor. She agreed, but mentioned that she would travel in her own carriage. The doctor insisted that she should travel in his private carriage. She refused, mindful of her reputation. The doctor kept pursuing her for months.

Haimabati often found herself ensnared in the corruption of her superiors. She describes 'a hair-raising incident' where a girl of eleven had been raped by her husband and was haemorrhaging. Haimabati was called to the house and found her unconscious. She asked the family to call the civil surgeon and the assistant surgeon, but despite their care the girl died. The rape of underage girls by their middle-aged husbands was common in those days. We have already discussed the 1889 case of Phulmoni Dasi, the ten-year-old Bengali girl whose rape and death at the hands of her thirty-five-year-old husband only resulted in a year's hard labour for the perpetrator. The case had shocked Bengali society and set the stage for the 1891 Age of Consent Bill, which made sex with a girl under twelve illegal, even if the perpetrator was her husband.

Thus, Haimabati knew that the husband was liable to be punished, but was powerless to do anything, while the civil surgeon wrote a certificate stating that the girl was fourteen and suffered septicaemia. He called Haimabati aside and asked her to say nothing, then gave her 500 rupees as her fee. Haimabati refused to take it but 'the surgeon shouted, "Why won't you take it? You have to." What could I do?' writes a hapless Haimabati. 'I took the money, but I was scared to death. What would my husband say? I would have to tell him and then everybody would find out what happened.'[241]

Haimabati tried to return the money and keep only 50 rupees, but the civil surgeon thought she was demanding more money, and he forced her to accept another 200 rupees. Haimabati now had to conceal the money from her husband. She kept it hidden in her clothes and doled it out to him little by little. The rest she spent on charity for a neighbouring family, buying them food, clothes and fruit.

This was the beginning of Haimabati's unusual charitable streak. 'I do not know if there is any virtue greater than charity,' Haimabati wrote. 'One may go in for lots of *pujas* and ritual observances, but I think charity is superior to all of these. One may ask "why do you resort to irregular ways?" But you well know women have no freedom. Even though men may be indifferent to material things, they are intensely worldly and have very little charity in their hearts.'[242]

By this time, Haimabati had two sons, and it was a struggle to balance the physically taxing work with home life. But she had no choice but to work, because the money she earned, 50 to 60 rupees a day, was the family's only income. The assistant surgeon Badrinath Mukherjee would repeatedly harass her, insisting that she travel in his carriage. The resourceful Haimabati found a way out—the Lady Dufferin Fund stipulated that no men could visit the offices or premises of the fund. She cited these rules to the civil surgeon, who banned Badrinath from visiting the Lady Dufferin Hospital. Then troubles of a different sort began. Every day Haimabati woke to find faeces smeared on her water pot, the pot for cooking rice, the door and the stairs. She would find faeces smeared on the doors and windows, and the carriage she used for travelling. The culprit could not be found.

Haimabati complained to the district magistrate, but the harassment did not stop.

All her life, her family had been a source of distress, not support, to Haimabati. This theme continued. Her brother-in-law, who had come to stay along with her younger sister, was a drunkard, and constantly tried to swindle money from her. Kunja Behari, always mindful of money, quarrelled with Haimabati and left the house.

One day, Haimabati saw two men slinking into the house. Terrified but resolute, she hit one on the head with her ruler. He turned out to be an associate of Badrinath Mukherjee. Haimabati heard from her staff that Mukherjee intended to kill her, and approached the civil surgeon, R.L. Dutt. Luckily for her, he was a Brahmo. The men were dismissed and things quietened down.

Mother, Other

Haimabati gave birth to a daughter, Bhakti Sudha, in 1896. By this time, the lack of help from Kunja Behari was getting to her. Her resentment was building. It all came to a head one day when Kunja Behari inexplicably gave her maids leave. Haimabati was suddenly summoned to an urgent case, and Kunja Behari was left with his baby daughter. This was unheard of. He shouted, 'You bastard woman, am I your father's servant? You want me to look after your daughter! I shall not permit this.' Haimabati blurted out, 'If you wish to live on your wife's income, then you will have to look after the children. I was not born with ten hands.'[243]

This was, of course, too much for Kunja Behari's fragile ego. He fell upon Haimabati 'like a bandit' and beat her mercilessly. Haimabati fell on a flower pot and cut her lip. Blood flowing profusely, Haimabati immediately fled to the civil surgeon's house and, unwisely blurted out that she could not work anymore. Her memoir is matter-of-fact, but her desperation is clear: she was simply at the end of her tether. Renouncing her beloved job was an act of utter frustration. Luckily for Haimabati, Dutt was not about to let her go so easily.

The Fighter

Dutt went to her house to plead with her husband, which quickly came to blows. Eventually Haimabati had to drag her husband away and lock him up. Poor Haimabati was deeply humiliated. It was exactly what Badrinath Mukherjee needed, and he lost no time in saying that Kunja Behari was negligent in not showing Haimabati her place. Haimabati was pressured to complain against her husband, but with three children, she could not do that.

Eventually, a compromise was reached. Haimabati was persuaded to stay apart from her husband, and he moved into separate lodgings in a nearby town. This should have been a relief for her, but her responsibilities only increased. Her second son was severely ill with a gastric complaint. She was told that he would not survive, and he did come very close to death's door for a month before eventually recovering. Her husband too was often ill.

It is typical of Haimabati's memoir that she spends very little time talking about her patients, and a lot of time talking about her family and their various illnesses. Simultaneously, she also berates them for not considering her weariness and fatigue. The picture that emerges, familiar to many women perhaps, is of a woman torn between her career and her family, sometimes beset with worry for them, at other times frustrated with their lack of consideration for her, the breadwinner, nurturer and all-round caregiver.

Haimabati had always been charitable, but visits to her husband's new residence made her even more so. She met children there who were so poor they would wait near dirty drains to drink the gruel thrown away from the rice 'of the babus'. They could afford to eat rice only once a month, and the rest of the time they would eat the greens, leaves and radishes they found in the fields.

Haimabati was deeply affected. She writes of the rapacious moneylenders who lent money to the poor at exorbitant rates, while the poor lived on leaves. This experience was to shape her life in the years to come.

Impact Of Lady Doctors In Bengal

Lady doctors from Campbell, such as Haimabati, were largely ignored by medical histories. But, by the end of the century, women trained in Western medicine were to be found in every district of Bengal.[244] These lady doctors, with VLMS licences, took medicine to remote areas where their better-educated, urban sisters would not go.

Contrary to expectations, most of the women did not drop out after their degrees. Haimabati worked as a doctor for over forty years. Another doctor, Musamut Idenessa, worked as the sole lady doctor of the Bidyamoyi Female Hospital in Mymensingh for twenty years.[245] Campbell lady doctors would not perform ambitious surgeries; rather, they would play a crucial role in delivering a hybrid form of medicine across rural Bengal.

Widowhood And A Houseful Of Children

Haimabati gave birth to two more sons, aided in the first labour by one of the many orphan children who hung around her house, as her husband was away. Then her husband became ill with diabetes. After a long period of illness, Kunja Behari died in 1902. They had been married for only thirteen years, but it must have seemed longer. Haimabati was left with five children, the oldest eight and the youngest only five months. She writes baldly, 'My duties increased a hundred-fold. I was both mother and father of our children as I no longer had anyone to depend on.'[246]

It was more important than ever for Haimabati to live frugally. But, with Kunja Behari gone, she succumbed to her charitable instincts, taking in a number of orphaned children of every religion. Before long, she was providing for thirty or forty children, most of whose mothers had died in her hospital. She would feed them by spreading a banana leaf on the floor, putting a ball of rice and lentils on it, then seating an older child next to a younger one and telling them to pretend that the younger one was their child—to eat first and then feed the child. She would leave the children to play and fight as she went on her rounds to the hospital, then return to bathe and feed them again.

Occasionally, she would send the children to other homes, but more would come in. Haimabati estimates that she cared for an astonishing 485 children, including day-old orphans.[247] Haimabati's life would certainly have been a lot easier if she had not had this constant and misplaced desire to mother orphans. By this time, people had begun sending older girls to her, and Haimabati would spend a great deal of money on their marriages, as much as 200 rupees per girl. Several were pregnant when they arrived, and she had to take care of their babies. Eventually, as her own sons grew up, she decided to stop taking in older girls and instead send them to other homes.

Haimabati lived for thirty-one years after the death of her husband, and her memoir in this period begins to get grimmer and grimmer. Her family proved to be an utter disappointment to her. She writes darkly of the 'harassment' she suffered from her daughter and sons, without revealing details. 'They did to me whatever they pleased,' she says. 'Everyone in this world whom I have been good to has mistreated me. No one has been just to me for a single day.'[248] Her sons managed to get good jobs, but Haimabati writes that none of them supported her. To be fair, all that piety and self-righteousness could not have been easy to live with—perhaps it was not easy for her family to support her charitable endeavours. She continued working until her last days, into her late sixties. Illness continued to dog her family, and

Haimabati paid the medical expenses for her grandchildren. In her last days, Haimabati grew ever more philosophical.

She wrote constantly of the need for women to work for the welfare of people, and not confine themselves to their families. Until the end, she remained deeply critical of regressive Hindu customs. She wrote of a Christian friend who married a Hindu man, that she was a highly qualified 'lady doctor'. But her education was wasted because 'her husband dolled her up like a housewife and confined her to the home out of regard for Hindu custom'. Haimabati was furious about the waste of talent and brains and remarked that even if her friend had worked two hours a day for the welfare of people, it would have done her a lot of good. 'I would be incapable of adjusting to such a life. I could not forget myself, forget God, give up my work and find peace in a few ornaments and fine clothes.'[249]

With her strong convictions and her disinclination towards the more feminine pursuits, Haimabati likely did not have many women friends. Her memoir is dominated by her friends amongst the Brahmos, but in the larger community she seems to have been isolated.

Why was Haimabati so unusual for her time? Professor Indrani Sen, from Sri Venkateswara College in New Delhi, who has studied Haimabati in detail, tells us why: 'First, she was a literate woman in an age when female literacy was taboo; second, she was a child-widow who remarried, with no family support, at the age of 23; third, she went through great difficulties and even dangers in her passion for learning; and lastly, she became a "lady doctor" and managed both *ghar* and *bahir* (home and outside) in her life. In all this she displayed a female subjectivity which was the driving force of her life.'[250] Haimabati was the classic example of a modern woman trying to have it all in a man's world. 'Discussing the issue of identity, one can also see, on her part, the appropriation of a "male" identity,' writes Indrani Sen. 'Indeed, there was a blurring of gender identities from her childhood itself, when she was affectionately nicknamed Chuni Babu (or "little mister Chuni") by her indulgent father. Equally "masculine" is the scientific temper and the tone of scientific scrutiny that she adopts.'[251] The only way Haimabati could make her way was to renounce emotion and be truly detached outwardly, like the men of her time, though inwardly she was furious.

Towards the end of her memoir, Haimabati writes of intense loneliness and an ever-constant preoccupation with domestic concerns, though she tried her best to withdraw from them. Her daughter's husband turned out to be a drunkard, and her youngest son was a wastrel.

'I have struggled and suffered all my life. What have I gained from all this? I have no companion but God,' she writes heartrendingly. Her memoir ends on 3 August 1933, with a long meditation on the divine. 'Great mother, blessed be your kindness, your mercy.'[252]

Two days later, on 5 August, the end came. She was sixty-seven. Her memoir would be stuffed into a trunk and forgotten, as would she. Eighty years later, it would finally be published. There is no franker or more unvarnished account of a lady doctor's life that survives from those times.

CHAPTER SIX

The Lawmaker

Muthulakshmi Reddy

'When father one day suggested to me that I would get a good salary as the headmistress of a local school, and that I might be satisfied with what little education I had, I ran to the well in the garden to put an end to my life. No offer of diamonds, no silk and money could tempt me away from my cherished desire.'

It was 1930. Quivering with nerves, a frail, bespectacled woman stood to address the Madras Legislative Council. She was forty-four, but called herself a 'babe legislator' because of her inexperience. She was only the second woman member of any legislature in India. Later, she would become the first woman in the world to become the vice president of a legislature. 'I had no other woman friend in the house to consult on that matter, and I must confess that I felt very nervous, with all eyes turned towards me, when I stood up to speak,' she would later write.[253] But stand she did. 'I am the only lady member in this assembly, even though one half of the population are women,' she said.[254]

Every Indian woman that exercises her right to vote, has Dr Reddy to thank (sometimes spelt Reddi by British writers). She was one of the main forces behind the long battle for universal franchise for Indian women. In a life full of incident, she would found India's premier cancer treatment institute and push legislation outlawing child marriage. The bill she was now nervously introducing sought to prevent the dedication of women to Hindu temples in the Madras Presidency.

In other words, to dismantle the devadasi system. Muthulakshmi was the daughter of a devadasi herself, though she kept this fact very quiet. Her mother, Chandrammal, came from the Isai Vellalar community, made up of artistes, music players and devadasis. (They are now classed as backward class).

A formidable section of the Hindu Brahmin orthodoxy stood against her on the bill. There was opposition from the powerful S. Satyamurti, a leading politician of the Indian National Congress, who would later become the mentor of K. Kamaraj, the eventual chief minister of Madras State. Satyamurti, a Brahmin, believed that the abolition of the devadasi system would eventually lead to the government interfering in Hindu customs and taking over temples. He argued that it deserved protection because it was a part of Hindu tradition.

Muthulakshmi would often find herself battling Hindu traditionalists. Nothing if not fearless, she had no patience for male hypocrisy and was not afraid of calling out men who preached against child marriage in public while they married off their young daughters in private.

She also sought to build up society; she set up institutions at a time when most foundations were established by the British. She founded the Adyar Cancer Institute and the Avvai Home and Orphanage for destitute girls. She began the first children's hospital in India: the Prince of Wales Hospital in Chennai.

We know about Muthulakshmi's life because she was one of the very few women of the time to actually write about herself. She wrote not one but two memoirs: *My Autobiography*, which covered her personal life, and *My Experience as a Legislator*. Both are invaluable accounts of the life of one of India's earliest professional working women. The picture that emerges from these memoirs is that of a single-minded, determined woman, who battled caste diktats and immense social pressure. Photographs of her show her with thick glasses and a uniformly earnest expression, looking much younger than her years.

But within her, many conflicts raged. Occasionally, though not often, her reserve would break down, and her frustration at being a woman in a man's world would reveal itself.

Breaking The Rules

Muthulakshmi was born Muthulakshmi Ammal, in the former princely state of Pudukkottai in Tamil Nadu on 30 July 1886. Her father, Narayanswami Iyer, was the headmaster of His Highness the Rajah's College, known as Maharajah College. He was a progressive man and Maharajah College a progressive institution, though still not progressive enough to allow women in.

Narayanswami, a Brahmin, was reportedly ostracised by his family for marrying a devadasi, yet it was Muthulakshmi's mother, Chandrammal, who was the more conservative and religious of the two.

Most of Muthulakshmi's childhood was spent battling her mother and aunts, who wanted to marry her off, in keeping with prevailing ideas that a girl unmarried after the age of ten, or puberty at the very latest, was unlucky. 'Sometimes the old women in our neighbourhood used to visit my mother and take her to task for keeping a daughter unmarried. My mother would weep over her fate for keeping an aged daughter in the family without marriage and feel very miserable.'[255] At ten, Muthulakshmi's marriage was arranged with a relative, but she had a lucky escape—one of her mother's sisters fell ill with consumption, and the wedding was cancelled.

After Muthulakshmi turned thirteen, with Narayanswami's support, she began to refuse all proposals of marriage. As young as she was, she had begun to see that leading the life of a conventional Indian woman was not for her. 'I had even then set my heart upon something high and I wanted to be a different woman from the common lot.'[256] Muthulakshmi was a rebel. Even as a child, she did not like going to noisy and crowded temples. This upset her mother, who blamed

Muthulakshmi's father for giving her an English education and apparently turning her into a Christian.

By now, Muthulakshmi, who suffered from asthma and bronchitis, showed signs of being both bright and remarkably ambitious. She had managed to wheedle her way into the local boys' school, which had better teachers than the girls' school. Despite the custom of girls being taught only Tamil, she coaxed the teachers into teaching her English. She was often teased and harassed by boys who saw her carrying her pile of books, but the young Muthulakshmi ignored them. She continued to walk alone.

The Prince And The Pauper

In 1902, Muthulakshmi passed the matriculation examination, one of the ten who passed from a hundred candidates, and of course, the only girl. 'The whole town was taken by surprise that a girl had beaten the boys in the examination and the boys smarted all the more under their failure,' wrote Muthulakshmi gleefully. She would always be intensely competitive, and enjoyed beating the boys.

It was then that Narayanswami realised her purpose and determination. He applied for her to join Maharajah College, despite it being only for men. The people of Pudukkottai were outraged. Never had a girl been educated beyond school. There was also opposition from the college, partly because of Muthulakshmi's gender, but also because of her caste. Most of the opposition came from conservative Brahmin men. Admitting her into a regular class would 'demoralise the boys', argued Radhakrishna Aiyar, the then principal of the college. A. Venkat Ramadoss, the dewan of Pudukkottai, observed, 'The policy of the state having all along been not to allow girls of the Melagar caste even into the sircar girls school (government girls school) in the town, and the furthering of the education of a girl of that caste not appearing to me to help the cause of female education in the state, I doubt that it is advisable.'[257] Muthulakshmi appealed to the raja of Pudukottai to help.

She was incredibly lucky that he was an unusual man, something of a maverick himself. Martanda Bhairava Tondaiman had a deep love for European culture. Born in 1875, he came to the throne at barely eleven, and was about twenty-seven when Muthulakshmi was entering college.

A juicy scandal was to come that would shock the town. In 1915, the raja would fall in love with Australian Molly Fink and marry her in Melbourne. A son, Martanda Sydney Tondaiman, would be born to them in 1916. Molly moved to India in 1915 and was presented to the gawping, fascinated citizens of Pudukkottai. But the British government refused to recognise her as the raja's wife, and accord her the privileges due to a rani. While in India, Molly almost died of vomiting and diarrhoea. On investigation, she was found to have been poisoned by the oleander plant, a traditional method of poisoning in the south. Martanda promptly left India with Molly and their son, and they spent the rest of their lives in Australia, and later in London and Cannes. Their son was also never recognised by the British government, and eventually he gave up his claim to the throne of Pudukkottai, to settle for a pension instead.

This then, was the man whom Muthulakshmi was appealing to, one not likely to follow the rules. He did not disappoint her. The raja passed an order that Muthulakshmi should be allowed to study in the college. To quote from the *Pudukkottai Gazette*, 'It must be said to the credit of the vision and independence of the Martanda Bhairava Thondaman, then Raja of Pudukkottai, that he overruled all objections and permitted her admission.'[258]

Muthulakshmi entered the college, the first woman to ever do so. When she joined, she was made to sit in a separate cordoned-off enclosure, invisible to the boys and visible only to the teacher. 'The boys would be curious to have a look at me and crowd around me wherever I went, though I always went about in a closed carriage. Some mischievous urchin boys would write anonymous letters and throw them into my room.'[259]

Her unusual dress made her stand out even more. Her father disliked her wearing a sari because he thought that educated women should dress differently from the rest, so she wore a skirt and coat with shoes. 'I must have looked funny indeed in that dress,' she said wryly, years later when she was called back to the Maharajah College, to address the students.[260]

Muthulakshmi went on to score high marks, passing her intermediate examination with distinction. Photos of the time show a frail young woman who seems barely able to stand. After her examination, she was found to be 'weak and anaemic', so she took a year off. During this time, her father taught her Shakespeare, Tennyson, Milton and Shelley. Muthulakshmi and her father would play badminton in their garden. This was against Pudukottai's strict social mores for girl children, who were meant to be confined to the home. 'The public of the state being unused to such treatment and liberties given to a girl would criticise my father,' wrote Muthulakshmi in her autobiography. 'Being a man of high principles and holding advanced views on women's education and respected by one and all in the state, he was able to hold his views against these criticisms.'[261]

Muthulakshmi had already studied further than any Pudukkottai girl. It now began to be suggested that she content herself with being a schoolteacher, an acceptable profession for women at the time. But she reacted strongly. When her father suggested that she would get a good salary as the headmistress of a local school, Muthulakshmi threatened to kill herself by jumping into the garden well. She would not settle for the commonplace.

Pudukkottai was too small to contain Muthulakshmi's ambition. And by sheer chance, another avenue opened up. A student of her father's, who was visiting Pudukkottai, asked if she had considered studying medicine at the Madras Medical College. At the time, there was still immense pressure on Muthulakshmi to marry, spearheaded by her mother, neighbours and the town in general. Muthulakshmi wanted to escape. As she said, with typical dry understatement, 'I wanted to get away from the place which was neither congenial nor helpful to my ideals.'[262]

At around this time, Muthulakshmi's mother fell ill with typhoid, rapidly becoming critical. So serious was her condition that family, friends and neighbours visited to say farewell. But by great good luck, an American doctor called Dr Van Allen was visiting the local hospital. Van Allen was a missionary who would later go on to establish the famous Van Allen Hospital in Kodaikanal, which still exists. Dr Allen was begged to treat her, and he prescribed treatment that effectively helped her recover. This incident, wrote Muthulakshmi, only made her more eager to become a 'medical woman'.[263]

Studying medicine was daunting. The course was gruelling, but she was prepared to take it on. It was also expensive. Once again, the raja of Pudukkottai helped out; he, along with other progressives, chipped in for the cost of her books and tuition.

Mingling In Madras

In 1907, Muthulakshmi and her father left for Madras. It was a heady time for the young girl. The city was at the height of its intellectual glory, teeming with nationalists, writers, poets and orators. And luckily for Muthulakshmi, she found herself surrounded by inspiring role models.

When she arrived in Madras, she was introduced to Dr M.C. Nanjunda Rao, by then already a legend in the city. Nanjunda Rao was the chemical examiner in Madras Medical College, a doctor to many zamindars and maharajas, and a nationalist who was a good friend of Annie Besant. With five sons, four daughters and sixteen horse carriages, Dr Rao lived a flamboyant life in Mylapore.

Among Rao's many exploits was helping the nationalist poet Subramania Bharati to escape arrest. Subramania Bharati was being tailed by the police and wanted to escape to Pondicherry. He hid out in Rao's huge house. Then, one night, Rao was rudely awakened in the middle of the night by the police, who had information that Bharati was concealed there. Rao convinced them that he was not harbouring a fugitive and sent them away. The Buckingham Canal ran past Rao's house. The next day he helped Bharati disguise himself as a fakir and arranged a boat to take him to Pondicherry.[264] Rao, who would visit Muthulakshmi's father and discuss politics, advised Muthulakshmi to give up medicine and take up journalism, but she did not listen.

Dr Rao's home was filled with the new breed of women, educated, brave, articulate, finding their own paths, completely different from the cloistered atmosphere of Pudukkottai. It was here that Muthulakshmi found her tribe, and she would spend the rest of her life making friends in these circles.

At Rao's house, Muthulakshmi met Sarojini Naidu, who made a huge impression on her. Sarojini Naidu's inter-caste marriage with Dr N.G. Naidu had taken place in Dr Rao's home, with his bless-ings. It was also at Dr Rao's home that Muthulakshmi met Ammu Swaminathan, who at only sixteen, was younger than her. The forceful, confident Swaminathan would go on to be a famous Gandhian, and serve as a member of the Constituent Assembly and the Rajya Sabha. Her famous family would include two incredible daughters: Captain Lakshmi Swaminathan, the celebrated freedom fighter who would join the Azad Hind Fauj, and Mrinalini Sarabhai, who became an accomplished and well-known dancer.

Swept up in this inspiring company, Muthulakshmi learnt to speak in public. She was often taken along to nationalist meetings to read speeches in Tamil. 'At about this time I accompanied Sarojini Naidu to a meeting at Adyar where Annie Besant spoke to a large audience under the banyan tree of Adyar, about the past glory of the Hindu period and the epic personalities of the Mahabharata and the *Ramayana*.' Muthulakshmi was powerfully moved by the feeling displayed by Besant. 'The audience was spellbound and her body shook with emotion when she spoke. My contact with all these great men and women and participation in some of these meetings was a very valuable experience to me.'[265]

Storming The Madras Medical College

The Madras Medical College (MMC) had a storied, progressive history. In 1865, it had admitted four women medical students, one British woman and the rest Anglo-Indian, at a time when most colleges in Europe and the US still barred women. Very little is known about three of the women, but the fourth was Mary Scharlieb (who has been mentioned earlier while speaking of Kadambini Ganguly's life, in Chapter 3). She entered MMC at the fairly advanced age of thirty.

At the time, many of the professors were against the admission of women. One professor told Scharlieb, 'I cannot prevent you walking around the wards, but I will not teach you.'[266] In 1878, the first Indian woman entered the MMC, Krupabai Satthianadhan. Unfortunately, a year later her health deteriorated, and she dropped out. She would go on to become a famous writer. By 1884, more women joined, including Abala Das, who would later marry biologist Jagdish Chandra Bose. Das would not practise, but would become an important social reformer, setting up a number of schools for women's education.

But the star of the MMC was undoubtedly Rose Govindarajulu, who would distinguish herself, getting a string of medical degrees from Edinburgh, Ireland and Brussels. She would then go on to serve the Mysore Medical Service for thirty-three years, retiring in 1920.[267]

Muthulakshmi thus had a number of women before her to show her the way, yet the road remained rough. Many professors, especially the British ones, continued to be prejudiced against female students. Nonetheless, Muthulakshmi managed to impress one of the most celebrated professors, Charles Donovan. He was the man who discovered the causative organism of kala-azar, which until then was called 'quinine-resistant malaria'. The parasite was named *Leishmania Donovani*, after Donovan and his partner Major Leishman.

Donovan was so taken with Muthulakshmi that he said, 'When she entered the hall to take her oral examination, she looked very nervous, but when the examiners started putting questions to her, out came the answers like bullets!'[268] Muthulakshmi also scored a perfect score in surgery, prompting another professor, Major Niblock, to announce her score in front of the class thus: 'A lady student, Muthulakshmi Ammal, has got a hundred per cent.'[269]

Another professor, the eccentric Maj. G.G. Gifford, famous for designing the maternity wing of the MMC—inaugurated in 1881—in the shape of a female pelvis, would also not allow female students to sit in his class.[270] And yet, Muthulakshmi won him over with her earnest demeanour and gained entry to the class.

In 1912, Muthulakshmi completed her five-year medical course, and graduated at the top of the class. She was the first Hindu woman to graduate from MMC. At a grand convocation, she was praised and fussed over, and her photo in the convocation gown was published in the papers. She joined the Government Hospital for Women and Children in Egmore as a house surgeon.

At the time, there were very few Indian women working as house surgeons. Muthulakshmi now had to give orders to European nurses and battle the innate racism of the Empire. The European nurses resented Indian women doctors, but Muthulakshmi convinced them of her ability, as she had done with numerous people before. In private, she commented sarcastically on the 'superiority complex of European nurses who used to address the Indian nurses as native midwives. Now after the National movement and the attainment of Independence, the appellation Native has been changed into Indian.'[271]

It was while she worked at the government hospital that Muthulakshmi found her second calling: social service for poor women and children. She joined a number of associations, including the Social

Service League of Madras and the Women's India Association, and also became a visiting doctor at the Young Widows Home in Egmore.

Family Life: A Mixed Bag

Muthulakshmi was a woman way ahead of her time. Despite her mother's desperation to get her married, she refused, worried that a husband would get in the way of her goals. She had a realist's view of marriage and how it benefited men while restricting women.

In her autobiography, she was outspoken about how marriage did not suit women. 'I did not want to become saddled with marriage and become subordinate to a man whomsoever he may be. I had seen in my place the ill-treatment accorded to wives by their husbands. So I did not want to be one of such victims of man's superiority and domination.'[272]

In 1912, staying unmarried was a radical move for a woman. But Muthulakshmi was determined to hold out for marriage on her own terms, or it would be no marriage at all. And in February 1913, along came a man who was willing to meet her halfway. Dr Sundara Reddy had heard glowing tales of Muthulakshmi's prowess from the professors at Madras Medical College. He wrote to her father with a proposal, which she at first rejected. Reddy then travelled to Madras to meet her, and after a few meetings, she agreed to marry him, but only if he promised to treat her as an equal. They were married in April 1914, with Brahmo Samaj rites. The bride was twenty-eight, nearly double the age of most brides of the time.

But marriage, even to a supposedly liberal man, was a rude shock for Muthulakshmi. Right away, she found herself pregnant. In 1915, she gave birth to their first son, Ram Mohan, after a traumatic pregnancy and birth. So traumatic, that she wrote in her autobiography, discreetly, 'As my husband and I did not want to go through another such childbirth, we swore that we would be only companions in life.'[273]

For years, the family was plagued with financial worries. Sundara

Reddy was the chief medical officer in Pudukottai, but was in debt because he had used his savings on his education. Muthulakshmi was the chief breadwinner, and right from the start, she continued her busy practice. Her memoirs describe the difficult life of a working mother. When her baby was only a month old, she was called to attend urgent cases because there were so few women doctors, especially for women in labour. Like so many working mothers, she felt constant guilt at not being able to be in two places at once. 'One evening I had to attend a difficult labour which required my constant attendance,' she wrote. 'My baby at home cried incessantly of hunger and would not drink any milk or sugar water as I was feeding the baby at that time. A messenger came to me but I could not leave the patient who was in a critical state. When I returned home, I found my own baby quite tired. However, I had the consolation that the patient whom I attended was found safe with her child.'[274]

Her son had many health problems, from diarrhoea to whooping cough, all described in detail in her memoirs. Every attack made Muthulakshmi more determined to help.

By this time, the family had moved back from Pudukkottai to Madras, an expensive city, where Muthulakshmi's income was much needed. And then, in 1918, 'in spite of our care', as Muthulakshmi delicately put it, she conceived again. Remembering her first difficult experience, Muthulakshmi employed Gifford, her professor and famous obstetrician, by then promoted to Lieutenant Colonel. The unplanned and initially unwanted baby, Krishnamurthi, would go on to become a famous doctor in his own right, the head of the Adyar Cancer Institute in Madras. He would work alongside his mother for many years, and be a great comfort to her.

Muthulakshmi had decidedly mixed feelings about the domestic sphere. There are hints in her autobiography that she did not find the institution of marriage as equal as she had been promised. Relations between the couple were strained, and they were beset by financial troubles, forcing Muthulakshmi to work when both children were still very young.

In her autobiography, she was frank, advising women doctors to not marry. 'Medical women, if they really love the profession and wish to practice, should not think of marriage, because they cannot perform two functions at one and the same time. As a mother I had to look after my delicate baby day and night, and as a wife I had to look after my domestic duties, and as a medical officer I had to do justice to my profession. I found it a great strain as well as a hardship to go through all these duties… Nobody could imagine the pain and suffering which a woman, especially a wife and a mother, nay an educated and economically independent woman, has to go through, especially when the husband is not very cooperative in the economy of the family.'[275]

By 1922, Muthulakshmi was earning 2,000 rupees a month, a huge sum in those days and nearly four times what her husband was earning as a professor of anatomy. She was the main breadwinner, a rare role for women of the time, and felt obliged to save money for the family, which was not well-off. This fact brought with it a feeling of accomplishment, but also immense stress and resentment.

It was at this time that something happened that deeply affected Muthulakshmi. She had always been close to her younger sister Sundarambal, who helped her in many ways with childcare and the household. Sundarambal, a teacher at a local college, suddenly took ill and it was found to be cancer of the rectum. At that time, cancer was thought to be fatal.

Muthulakshmi tried her best to save her sister, sending her to Calcutta and Ranchi for radium treatment, and nursing her lovingly. As Muthulakshmi wrote in her autobiography, 'She would sit and pray in the nights for hours together for her relief (sic) from her tortures. She suffered for almost a year. I had to inject morphia three or four times a day. It left an indelible impression on my sensitive mind. Ever after, I was bent upon finding a remedy for this human scourge.'[276]

Sundarambal's painful death would change Muthulakshmi's life, but it would also, one day, change the lives of millions.

Blighty And More Tragedy

In 1925, Muthulakshmi was offered a scholarship by the Government of India to study the diseases of women and children in the UK. To give up her lucrative practice was a hard decision, but Muthulakshmi was determined to learn more about the subject that consumed her: cancer. Sundarambal's agonising death had made her determined to explore cures for the disease.

With Muthulakshmi travelled her two sons, aged eleven and six, and her husband. Her memoir has a comical paragraph about her travelling arrangements. 'I always carried with me a metal *kooja* (jug) of water and brass tiffin box. The French Porter in Marseilles, not used to such articles held them upside down with the result that everything dropped down on the floor to the annoyance of Dr Reddy, who always objected to my carrying these vessels with me. As our *kooja* water was not available the children became very thirsty. We had to purchase Vichy bottled water at Rs 1 per bottle to quench our thirst. This gave me an opportunity to bring home to Dr Reddy the value of our Indian *kooja*!'[277] A picture emerges of a frugal woman who always had to have the last word, annoying though that might have been to others.

England was a revelation for Muthulakshmi, especially with regard to the British way of managing hospitals and treating diseases that people would have died of in India. She had an operation of the cervix in Chelsea hospital, to guard against cervical cancer, and was lavish in her praise. Chelsea was a voluntary hospital managed by the British public. 'We have yet to learn much from the British in the way of managing hospitals. The English people gave ample financial support to their hospital. I found English people a well-disciplined race with a strong civic sense.'[278]

She also had company in London. Muthulakshmi's sister

Nallamuthu was already in the city, studying at the London School of Economics. Nallamuthu was something of a genius in her own right. She would later go on to become the first Indian woman president of the Queen Mary College in Chennai.

When Muthulakshmi had been only a month in the UK, tragedy struck again. Her only brother, an advocate in the high court, passed away. Muthulakshmi considered returning to India, but once again, her steely nature won. She writes, 'I could not bring my brother back to life.' She stayed on to learn more.

Paris And Public Life

For some time, Muthulakshmi had been craving a larger canvas for her many talents. And in 1926, on her way back from London, she got the chance to enter public life. The Women's India Association asked Muthulakshmi to represent them as a delegate at the First International Congress of Women in Paris; women from forty-two countries would be attending the conference.

Muthulakshmi's speech focused on the ancient rights of Indian women, whom she saw as emancipated. 'There are examples of illustrious Indian women in the past who had distinguished themselves in every sphere of life... such as the famous Padmini of Rajputana, Chandbibi the warrior queen, Kaikeyi of the *Ramayana* and the famous Avvai of the Tamil country whose immortal verses will live so long as the world lasts.'[279] Muthulakshmi, ever a fervent nationalist, blamed the current subordinate position of women on foreign invasions and internal dissension.

The Congress was important for Muthulakshmi's development in other ways. For the first time, she began to see the interests of women as different from men. She thought that the best way to have women's interests represented was to have more women in public life. This was revolutionary even for Western women, much less an Indian woman brought up to be dependent on men. After the conference, Reddy wrote that 'women suffer persecution, injustice and inequality of treatment', and that women's interests are different from those of men whose selfishness and claim to superiority 'inflict many hardships on women.'[280]

This was also the time when Muthulakshmi became deeply influenced by Gandhian ideals, for better or for worse. She was to carry on a prolonged correspondence with Mahatma Gandhi, over such issues as child marriage, votes for women and the abolition of the devadasi practice.

But all this was yet to come. In the meantime, a debate close to Muthulakshmi's heart began to gain prominence: the universal franchise for women.

Who Gets To Vote?

The fight for the right to vote for Indian women began in 1917. Initially, it was spearheaded by British suffragettes who had come to India. They would discover that Indian women would have their own ways of doing things, rooted in their own culture.

By the time the Indian campaign began, British suffragettes had already been fighting for the vote for women for over a decade. They began with peaceful demonstrations and petitions. But when their demands were not met, they took to violent means. By 1912, their leader Emmeline Pankhurst and other radical suffragettes had taken to arson, window smashing, assaulting police officers and eventually, bombings. Soon, nearly a thousand suffragettes had been imprisoned.

Their demands for universal franchise had been met with derision; the suffragettes were heckled and even pelted with eggs. There was a popular song that hecklers would sing at women's meetings:

> Put me on an island where the girls are few
> Put me with the most ferocious lions in the zoo
> Put me in a prison and I will never ever fret
> But don't put me near a Suffering-gette.[281]

But the 'Votes for Women' campaign in India was very different. In general, Indian women were law-abiding, content to present memorandums and testify before committees. Indian women wanted to fight alongside men, not *against* them. Besides, Indian women like Muthulakshmi still believed that the most important battle was against colonialism and the British Empire, not their own countrymen. Independence first, rights for women later.

In 1917, the Women's India Association was begun by the theosophist Annie Besant, Dorothy Jinarajadasa and the Irish activist Margaret Cousins. Jinarajadasa and Cousins had been radical feminists in the UK, but in India they were influenced by theosophy, and tailored their methods to suit Indian women. They were joined by the mercurial Sarojini Naidu. That same year, an All-India Women's deputation of fourteen women leaders from all over the country, led by Sarojini Naidu, presented a memorandum to E.S. Montague of the Montague-Chelmsford Commission, demanding that women be given voting rights.

As ahead of their time as these women were, they still saw women as helpmeets and companions to men. Politics was seen as the domain of men, and women would bring a softer, gentler, kinder aspect to it. The word 'mother' was used often, and much reference made to the nurturing qualities of women. At the 1918 Congress session, Naidu spoke for many of her peers when she reassured, 'We ask for the vote not that we might interfere with you in your official functions, your civic duties, your public place and power, but rather that we might lay the foundation of national character in the souls of the children that we hold upon our laps.'[282]

There was also dissension in the Women's India Association over the reservation of seats for women. Muthulakshmi was way ahead of her fellow leaders in this. Unlike her peers, she was suspicious of men's motivations and 'cautioned against placing too much faith in male gratitude'. But the majority of women in the association and outside of it, were not in favour of reservations, for fear of seeming too forward and encouraging communal reservations. This would have serious impact later, when women representatives would be elbowed out of politics.

In 1919, the South Borough Franchise Committee visited India to study the matter of voting rights, and then recommended that women should be totally excluded from the franchise. The committee argued that Indian women were still uneducated and held back by social mores, and that giving them the right to vote would have to wait for more than a few years.

The Women's India Association was furious. Besant warned that Indian women would join their men in fighting against the British, if they were ignored. Sarojini Naidu argued angrily that Indian women had come a long way and were qualified enough to vote.

A compromise was reached. The Government of India Act Bill, 1919 passed on the responsibility to the provinces, but allowed them to enfranchise only select, elite women with incomes and property. It did not allow women to stand in elections.

In 1921, Madras became the first province in India to allow women to both vote and stand for elections. The Bombay Presidency followed a few months later. But the right to vote was still only limited to married women who owned property, and on the basis of their husband's qualifications.

Even this limited franchise was unpopular. A reader from Saidapet in Madras wrote a letter to the editor, where he exclaimed, 'It is not a matter of congratulations that the legislative council should have resolved to extend suffrage to Indian women. For progress, man must be both the controller in politics and civics. His sex stands for performance, conformity and therefore, for uniformity, essential for common good and justice.'[283]

To her credit, Muthulakshmi strongly opposed the property condition. 'We women wish to be citizens in our own rights, independent of any of our male relations,' she wrote in her autobiography. She adds, 'We do not think that women's rights as a citizen should depend upon her marriage, which in the majority of cases in India at present, is not entirely under her control.' She also includes an element of social justice, as she says, 'We do not wish that the votes of the propertied class should be doubled by giving the vote only to the wife of the properly qualified man, as it will place the poor labouring class at a disadvantage.'[284] But her opposition was of no use. The right to vote continued to be restricted to those elite who owned property.

Thereafter, women began to be appointed to legislatures. Travancore was the first Indian state to appoint a woman to the representative assembly, Mary Poonen Lukose (more on her later in Chapter 7). Madras was the second, and the woman it appointed was Muthulakshmi, in 1927. When Muthulakshmi was nominated to the legislature, she was initially reluctant to take office. Giving up her medical career to enter politics was a huge step, especially when there were so few women in politics, and those who were in it were often mere figureheads. She was inspired by Gandhi's writings, where he pushed for more women to join the nationalist movement. In 1930, when Gandhi was arrested after the Dandi Salt March, Muthulakshmi would resign from the legislature in protest.

The kind of woman voter that the early women in politics envisaged was a respectable, educated wife and mother. There was no room for prostitutes or the uneducated, and in the end 'neither opponents nor proponents of reservations were interested in bringing women unlike themselves into politics.'[285] Muthulakshmi herself argued that 'women of character, grit and courage should be chosen to occupy places of honour and responsibility'. In reality, this meant Gandhian women from elite backgrounds, with husbands by their sides.[286] It would take until 1950 for women to win universal adult franchise, and for every woman—rich, poor, single or married—to have the vote.

Muthulakshmi On Men

Was Muthulakshmi a feminist? If she was, it was not the kind we know today. Indeed, she believed that Indian men were mostly supportive of the women in their lives.

In *My Experiences as a Legislator*, she wrote that she had two objects in writing the book. 'The one is to show such of my sisters and others who still hold the view that women are created only for the home and men for the state, how women's activity could be profitably extended from the home to the city.' She was clearly against the confinement of women to the home. But her other object was more singular. 'To demonstrate to the outside world how much Indian men honour and respect their women colleagues.'[287]

In 1947, when India achieved independence, Muthulakshmi would write an editorial in *The Hindu*. Once again, she blamed outside influences for the current low status of women, this time, the Mughal invasion. 'In the early history of India the women walked the earth the equals of men. But the foreign invasion, a thousand years ago, drove them into a long exile. They had to face men who neither spared life nor honour. And in adapting themselves to a changing environment they passed into purdah and the burning pyre, into seclusion and the backyard of history.'

In the editorial, she praised Annie Besant and women's associations for their work, but reserved the bulk of her appreciation for men. She lavishly praised men, from Raja Ram Mohan Roy to Dayanand Saraswati and Ishwar Chandra Vidyasagar for 'freeing women from the bonds and customs and conventions that hampered their growth physically and mentally'.

Reddy distanced herself from the suffragettes by arguing that Indian women had always had rights; they had just been forgotten and buried. 'The political and social emancipation movements of the women of India lacked the drama and struggle of the western suffragettes. Because it was not the coming for the first time to a new

consciousness of the ideals of service,' she argued, 'but only as re-awak-
ening and re-kindling of that consciousness… in the minds of men
of India who had never by word or deed put any difficulties in the
way of the women of India, or obstacles in the way of their claims for
advancement and emancipation.'[288]

It is interesting that Muthulakshmi seemed to have forgotten the
many men who had indeed put obstacles in the way of women, including S. Satyamurti and the men who opposed her various legislations.
Perhaps, after the years of struggle for Independence, she was in a
mood for reconciliation.

And yet, despite this conciliatory line, Muthulakshmi was no
pushover. She would carry on a long feud against the formidable C.
Rajagopalachari, the last governor general of India, and the second
chief minister of Madras State. In 1937, Muthulakshmi was invited
to stand for the legislature by both the Congress and the Justice party,
which was a party founded to give non-Brahmins representation. She
chose to contest as a Congress candidate, only to be eventually denied
a party ticket by Rajagopalachari and her old foe S. Satyamurti.

She would write scathingly of him, 'Though Rajaji is a great politician and sacrificed much for the country's freedom, in my opinion, he
is a reactionary in regard to social reforms, particularly in the emancipation of women. He believes the ancient customs and practices, and
is not for any change.'[289] In 1952, Rajaji became the chief minister of
Madras state. By then, Muthulakshmi had won a reputation as a social
reformer. More women had joined government as well. Rajaji found
himself in need of a female legislator, and he asked Muthulakshmi
to join the Madras Legislative Council. She was sixty-seven by then,
and at first declined, but then accepted after wheedling a plot of land
for her cancer hospital out of him. Muthulakshmi was nothing if not
canny and adaptable.

The Handmaidens Of The Gods

In 1927, the crusading Muthulakshmi came up against a formidable opponent. Her adversary was a woman, who in her own way was as much of a stubborn pioneer as Muthulakshmi. This was Bangalore Nagarathnamma, a devadasi who was born into poverty, and eventually became a highly respected musician, successfully fighting for women to perform at the annual Carnatic music celebration, Thyagaraja Aradhana.

To understand the tussle between Nagarathnamma and Muthulakshmi, it is necessary to first understand the complicated history of the devadasis. As mentioned earlier, Muthulakshmi herself was the daughter of a devadasi. But she does not mention this in either of her autobiographies. 'She never mentioned being from the devadasi community, and neither did her son,' says Dr V. Shanta, chairperson of the Cancer Institute (WIA), who worked for many years with Muthulakshmi's son Dr S. Krishnamurthi. 'I can only surmise it was because of the stigma. I wish she had talked about it.'[290] One can hardly blame Muthulakshmi, given how she was initially denied entry into college because of her caste. In contrast, Nagarathnamma was fiercely proud of being a devadasi.

The word 'devadasi' means 'handmaiden of the gods', and when the practice began, girls of all castes could be dedicated to the gods.[291] Devadasis were often well educated and literate at a time when other women were not. Those who could sing or dance were trained to a high level; the rest performed duties such as cleaning and looking after the deity in the temple. The devadasis had many privileges. They had a right to the property bequeathed to them by the temple, and property passed from mothers to daughters, in sharp contrast to the rest of society. The birth of a girl was welcomed.

There is no firm record of when the practice first began, but an inscription in the Brihadeeswara temple dating from the time of

Raja Raja Chola, who ruled from 985 to 1013 AD, states that four hundred dancing girls were appointed for temple service. Most significantly, it orders that land be given to these women, which consisted of the 'produce of one *veli* of land, a hundred *kalam* of paddy.'[292]

When they died, their descendants who were qualified would receive the same allowance. The devadasi practice continued during the Vijaynagar empire and the Marathas, with the devadasis being highly respected by rulers who appreciated the beauty of the arts. They were not considered prostitutes, though they could take lovers.

But by the 19th century, devadasis had begun to fall on hard times. Temples began to lose their prominence and power, and devadasis were forced to perform for wealthy landlords, princes and officials. In 1792, a French priest, Abbe Jean-Antoine Dubois, visited India, and reported on the by then pitiable decline of the devadasis. Dubois had, of course, a puritan, Victorian and colonialist point of view. Nevertheless, his account is useful.

Dubois wrote of the decline in temple earnings, which forced the devadasis to turn to prostitution. 'The devadasis receive a fixed salary for the religious duties which they perform, but as the amount is small, they supplement it by selling their favours in as profitable a manner as possible. All the time which they have to spare in the intervals of the various ceremonies is devoted to infinitely more shameful practices; and it is not an uncommon thing to see even more sacred temples converted into mere brothels.'[293]

By the late 19th and early 20th century, as temple patronage had almost completely collapsed, opinion on devadasis was sharply divided. Were they prostitutes or custodians of the arts? Perhaps a bit of both.

The author and music historian V. Sriram sums it up. 'Though it is fashionable today to think of all devadasis in highly romantic terms, they were in reality a community of women who were exploited by men, and then abandoned when they were no longer of any use. Finding patrons for their daughters was the main occupation for many devadasis, and most of them were considered to be hard-nosed grabbers who were out to milk their patrons, bringing untold sorrow to the legitimate wives and families. On the one hand the community was the storehouse of the arts. On the other, it was the repository of all evil, and every conceivable vice.'[294]

It was in this atmosphere that Nagarathnamma was born in November 1878, into a devadasi family in Mysore. When the baby was a year old, her mother Puttulakshmi had a fight with her patron Subba Rao, and both mother and child were thrown out of his house. Such was the precariousness of the devadasi life. Puttulakshmi was determined to give her daughter a secure life, and Nagarathnamma received a thorough education, in music, dance and several languages—Kannada, Tamil, Telugu and even English.

The young Nagarathnamma moved to Madras, then the centre of music and dance. By 1905, she had become so successful that she had bought a house of her own, had a huge stash of jewellery and was paying her own income tax. With society's increasing disapproval of dance performances, she gave up dancing and focused on music, and with her knowledge of Sanskrit, also began religious discourses. She was as respectable as it was possible for a devadasi to be.

Then, in 1910, Nagarathnamma shocked the polite society of Madras by editing a book by Muddhu Palani. Palani was a court poetess and concubine of Pratapsimha, a Maratha ruler who ruled Thanjavur from 1739 to 1763. Like Nagarathnamma, Muddu Palani was proud of her learning; she wrote *Radhika Santwanamu* (The Appeasement of Radha), which was about the erotic passion of Radha for Krishna.

Muddu Palani's identity was so erased that in later years people thought she was a man. Later, the Andhra reformer Kandukuri Veeresalingam Pantulu, who believed that devadasis were reprehensible, called Muddu Palani an adulteress and pronounced the work to be shameful. In a frenzy of puritanism, Veerasalingam declared that anything written by a prostitute could only be shameless and unsuitable for women to read, and called it 'bereft of the modesty that one expects from a woman.'[295]

The unapologetic Nagarathnamma, always deeply proud of her heritage, was not having any of this hypocrisy. Was modesty a virtue only applicable to women, she asked, pointing out that Veeresalingam had edited works written by men with far more graphic descriptions. Such terms as chastity, according to her, did not apply to devadasis.[296]

Nagarathnamma's actions were incredibly brave for her time. To be proud and unashamed of being a devadasi, to stand up against a powerful man like Veeresalingam and to speak for the right of women to write anything they wanted, was unprecedented. Her defence of the book stirred up a debate. In January 1911, the Telugu paper *Sasilekha* attacked the book: 'A prostitute composed a book under the name of Radhika Santwanam and then another prostitute corrected errors therein and edited it.'[297]

A case for obscenity was registered against the book, and several other books considered racy. Nagarathnamma and the publisher, Venkata Ranga Rao, defended the book on the grounds of literary merit. Rao argued that the books were classics, but to no avail.

Eventually, copies of *Radhika Santwanamu* were seized, and future copies were expurgated. But the entire episode made Nagarathnamma a force to reckon with in the world of literature as well as music.

Soon she would take another courageous step: one that would lead to her being forever linked to Thyagaraja, the greatest of Carnatic music composers. Thyagaraja had died in 1847, after renouncing the world and becoming a saint. Ever since his death, various warring factions of devotees had celebrated an annual aradhana, or ceremony of adoration. The various factions were united on one thing though—no woman could participate. This was exactly the kind of prejudice that enraged Nagarathnamma, who was an ardent devotee of Thyagaraja.

Nagarathnamma's concerts had made her even more wealthy, and she was not afraid to use her money. She built a temple for Thyagaraja near his samadhi in Thiruvaiyaru. Then she went further: launching a separate concert that women were allowed to participate in. Eventually Nagarathnamma's concert became more popular than the one organised by the leading factions. In 1941, it was decided to hold one annual concert. Today, five times more women than men sing at the Thyagaraja festival, held annually in Chennai.[298]

This then was the doughty woman whom Muthulakshmi would battle, a woman who was as rooted and respected in her own community as Muthulakshmi was in hers. But by 1927, the tide of opinion was against the devadasis. Social reformers, Christian missionaries and Gandhians were against the practice, and most considered devadasis to be no different from prostitutes. Muthulakshmi tabled her resolution in the legislative council to ask the Madras government to end the dedication of women to temples.

The resolution took the devadasi community by surprise. They had not expected legal action. Muthulakshmi wrote, 'I have been feeling all along and feeling most acutely too that it was a great piece of injustice, a great wrong, a violation of human rights, a practice highly revolting to our higher nature to countenance, and to tolerate young innocent girls to be trained in the name of religion to lead an immoral life, to lead a life of promiscuity, a life leading to the disease of the mind and the body.'[299] Muthulakshmi was supported by Gandhi, who wrote in *Young India*, 'The devadasi system is a blot upon those who countenance it. It would have died long ago but for the supineness of the public. I am therefore of the opinion that Muthulakshmi's proposal is no way premature. Such legislation might well have been brought earlier.'[300]

Muthulakshmi wrote that her attempt to abolish the devadasi system 'had the cordial support of all sections of the people'. In this, she was being disingenuous at best, deceptive at worst. Nagarathnamma and other devadasis objected to the move to pass this resolution, and registered their protest at being clubbed with prostitutes. They wrote a memorandum titled 'The Humble Memorandum of the Devadasis of the Madras Presidency' and sent it to C.P. Ramaswami Aiyar, the law member of the Government of Madras. They acknowledged that a few members of the community 'had strayed', but all devadasis could not be condemned. Finally, they argued that the proposed law would only increase prostitution, and that they would be thrown into the 'very jaws of hunger, despair and prostitution' and deprived of their source of living.[301] Instead, they asked for gradual evolution, and the recognition of out-of-wedlock arrangements with their patrons.

Protest meetings were held in many towns of the Madras Presidency. Nagarathnamma played a prominent role, attending meetings, signing many letters of protest and approaching influential people. As always, in Madras, the matter was thoroughly discussed in the columns of *The Hindu*. Muthulakshmi wrote a fervent letter in the newspaper, dated 15 November 1927, defending her position. '95% of devadasis lead a life of prostitution and the remaining 5% take to a life of concubinage... In this unfortunate land,' argued Muthulakshmi, 'every kind of evil goes under the cloak of religion and custom, which state of things is the chief and true cause of our ill health, poverty and dependent position in the world.'[302]

Despite Muthulakshmi's good intentions, the devadasi women became scapegoats for the sins of men. In December 1927, the All India Music Conference was held, comprising musicians from across India. In his speech, the conference president Dr U. Rama Rau admitted the contribution of devadasis to the art form. 'If today South Indian music is not dead and its glowing embers kept alive, it is due partly if not wholly to the devadasi community, to whom we must acknowledge our gratitude,' he said. But he then went on to shame them for 'their unpardonable sins for whom they now stand arraigned before the public forum.'[303] No mention was made of the role men played in their situation.

In recent times, Muthulakshmi's stance has been seen by some as patronising and elitist. Muthulakshmi was firm in her conviction that only educated, 'respectable' women such as herself could speak on behalf of the devadasis, or indeed participate in public life. She was contemptuous of the efforts made by Nagarathnamma and others to discuss this immensely complicated issue and constantly repeated that the devadasis were victims of tradition, ignorant of healthy living and trained only to lead an immoral life.

Her sniffy dismissal of the devadasis' concerns may have been indicative of how deeply she wanted to flee her own roots. When her old classmate from Maharajah College,

K. Satyamurti, who had also joined politics, argued in the legislature that abolishing the devadasi system would result in temples and traditional arts being taken away from the Hindus, Muthulakshmi responded, quick as a shot, 'Let Brahmin girls take up the duty then, since the devadasis have done it for so long.'[304] It was an argument hard to refute.

And indeed, this is exactly what happened. It took some years for the Devadasi Act to be passed, because of opposition from Hindu conservatives. By the early '50s, the last of the cultured and trained devadasis had died out. The dance tradition of the devadasis was appropriated by Brahmin women, in the guise of Bharatanatyam. The danseuse Rukmini Devi Arundale set up Kalakshetra in Chennai to make dance 'respectable' again and rescue it from its sleazy reputation. Bharatanatyam was reborn as a respectable and conservative dance form, but the devadasis were no longer its guardians.

Nagarathnamma spent the last years of her life in silent communion with Thyagaraja, singing his songs. The end came in 1952. She was buried near Thyagaraja's samadhi, the first time that Thiruvaiyaru allowed the burial of a woman. By then, Muthulakshmi had gone on to greater glories.

The Fight To Abolish Child Marriage

Muthulakshmi now threw herself into a bigger challenge: the abolition of child marriage.

Opposition to child marriage had been building up in the liberal community since the days of Anandibai and Rukhmabai. The Age of Consent Act had been passed in 1891, but that only prohibited consummation of marriages with young girls, and not the actual marriage. The few Indian women in public life—all of them liberal and educated—began to emphasise the need for a more comprehensive law. There was strong opposition from Hindu orthodox men, however, so the British government thought it most expedient to stay out of the matter.

By 1927, the reformers had had enough of prevarication. That year, Rai Harbilas Sarda, a legislator from Rajasthan, introduced a bill that suggested raising the age of consent from thirteen to fourteen in the case of married girls, and fourteen to sixteen in the case of unmarried ones. It also suggested a very bold step: invalidating all marriages below this minimum age. It applied only to Hindus, Sikhs and Jains.

Women's organisations thought this altered age of consent still too low. An All India Women's Conference was held in Pune for the first time in 1927, at which they recommended a minimum age of marriage of sixteen for girls and twenty-one for boys, though they must have known that it would never be accepted.

The All India Women's Conference urged that Muslims and other communities should also be restrained from underage marriages. Delegations of women met Mohammad Ali Jinnah, Madan Mohan Malviya, Motilal Nehru and Lajpat Rai, among others, to demand a strong law applicable to all. After much discussion, the Sarda Bill resulted in the Child Marriage Restraint Act, popularly known as the Sarda Act of 1929, which prescribed the minimum age for marriage of boys as eighteen and that of girls as fourteen years, two whole years below what women demanded.

Even this was a tough pill to swallow for conservative men of all religions. A powerful section of Indian men argued that the Act should not apply to them as it would interfere with their personal law. Besides, they argued disingenuously, child marriage was not common amongst Muslims.

But Muslim women hit back. In a speech at the All India Women's Conference session in 1928, the begum of Bhopal condemned child marriage, saying that it was 'incumbent upon us to stop this evil, as far as possible'. Child marriage, she argued, was prevalent amongst all communities.

It is hard to explain, almost a century later, just how significant and difficult this was in 1928. This was the first time women were speaking out in the public sphere and debating issues that affected them; and it was the first time men were forced to let women talk, for lack of other options. The women's conference members gathered all their courage to stand up to religion, patriarchy and hundreds of years of deeply entrenched custom.

Meanwhile, Muthulakshmi was preparing her own assault. In 1927, she introduced her own bill against child marriage in the legislature. We have no way of knowing, because she does not mention it in her biography, but perhaps the debate over child marriage was deeply personal; perhaps it brought back her own childhood, forever evading attempts to be married off before twelve, and fighting to study.

Whatever her motivation, she did not hold back from attacking religion, custom and respectable Hindu men in her defence of the bill. 'Every social evil in this blessed country goes in the name of religion. What is custom after all?' she asked. 'If any practice is observed for a few years owing to the exigencies of the times, it becomes sanctified as a custom. So, let not the government be frightened into inaction by the cry that religion is in danger.'[305]

Muthulakshmi scornfully dismissed the argument that gradual education and reform would eventually make a difference, without laws. 'We have been doing effective propaganda work all these fifty or sixty years, and still the progress is very little. I have now figures on hand to show that early marriages are rather on the increase through-out India.'[306]

Muthulakshmi was also unafraid to take on the hypocrisy of Hindu conservative men, especially those who preached reform outside and were deeply regressive inside their own homes. Her impatience at their bigotry was scorching. 'If the government could ask us to wait until every parent is educated, I am afraid we will have to wait until the Doomsday, because I know that the very same gentlemen who preach against the early marriage on the platform, on return home forget all about it and practice early marriage in their own family. Preaching is one thing and practicing is quite another thing,' she wrote.[307]

Muthulakshmi also had no hesitation in taking on Gandhi. At the time, Gandhi, and many in the nationalist movement, were of the view that achieving Swaraj or independence, was important above all things, and that social reform could come later. Gandhi himself had been married at the age of only thirteen to his wife Kasturba, and was staunchly against child marriage. But he still thought reforms could wait. In May 1928, Muthulakshmi wrote a three-page letter to Gandhi, urging him to make an unequivocal statement against child marriage.

'If the members of the Congress believe that freedom is the birth right of every individual, should they not first liberate their women from the evil customs and conventions that restrict their all-round healthy growth?' She did not let it rest there. 'Would you kindly advise our men to follow the right and surest way to freedom?' she badgered. Gandhi replied tersely, 'I have your letter. I agree with you that there is no salvation for men without women's salvation. I assure you that I miss no opportunity of driving the truth home to men.'[308]

Gandhi later wrote in *Young India,* 'I am strongly in favour of raising the Age of Consent not merely to 14, but even to 16. Sanskrit texts of doubtful authority cannot be invoked to sanctify a practice which is itself immoral. But I am painfully conscious of the fact that even the existing legislation has proved abortive for want of public opinion to support it. The task before the reformer in this is most difficult.'[309]

A Home For The Forgotten

In the mid-1930s, Muthulakshmi began thinking about alternative ways in which young girls who had been in the devadasi system could support themselves. She also wanted to set up a halfway house for them.

Muthulakshmi's son, Krishnamurthi, recalled how the Avvai Home was founded. He was a boy of ten and playing in the courtyard when two young girls approached him saying they had come to meet his mother. 'They began to weep when they saw her and explained that they were two sisters from the devadasi community who had refused "dedication", and having nowhere else to go, came to her seeking help and protection. The next day my mother sent the girls to what was known as the "Non-Brahmin hostel" in Triplicane for admission. When they came back weeping, denied admission on the grounds of being from the devadasi community, my mother was aghast! She told me they were my new sisters and were going to stay.'[310]

In the Madras of that era, shelter homes were separate for Brahmins and non-Brahmins. The Avvai Home was the first to allow girls of any religion, caste or creed. In those days, this was radical. Initially, it only took in devadasi girls, but then it began to take in all orphans and destitute girls. The home was managed by Muthulakshmi's sister, Nallamuthu Ramamurthi.

Today, the Avvai Home is a Chennai institution. It provides education for more than nine hundred girls, runs a government-aided school and houses a teacher-training institute. As for the two devadasi sisters, one grew up to become a teacher and the other a nurse.

'Why A Cancer Hospital? People Only Die Of Cancer.'

For over forty years, Muthulakshmi had carried with her the memory of her sister's painful death from rectal cancer. She had been unable to do anything back then, but the idea of doing something for cancer patients had never left her.

She began as early as 1935, but her efforts were side-lined, and then World War II obliterated all other concerns. When the war years were over, she began to think of a cancer hospital again, but she needed an ally. By then, her husband had passed away. She decided that her supporter would be her second son, S. Krishnamurthi. He was sent to the US to study medicine in 1947, even though the family had very little money. Muthulakshmi sold her car and whatever property she had to fund him. Krishnamurthi called this ambitious plan 'Operation Cancer'.[311]

He returned two years later, very reluctantly. Krishnamurthi had got more experience in the UK, and landed a job at the Royal Free Hospital in London. He was all set to begin work there when he got a telegram from his mother. 'Seriously ill!' said the telegram, and the good doctor rushed back. He found his mother perfectly well. She said, calmly, 'I sent you abroad to study so that you could come back and serve our people, not live comfortably in a foreign country.'[312] Krishnamurthi understood the message.

To begin with, Krishnamurthi had little desire to help his patriotic mother in what seemed then to be a hopeless cause. 'I had no enthusiasm for her missionary zeal, nor any inclination to be a heroic pioneer triumphing over odds and ordeals.' Eventually, Muthulakshmi stopped talking to him of service to humanity, and explained the heartbreak she had personally suffered when her sister was diagnosed with cancer. Her dream to work towards finding a cure for the disease would be shattered if he did not help, she said. 'Mother and son had a very strong bond,' explains Dr Shanta.[313] Krishnamurthi decided to join Muthulakshmi in her fight, a decision that would change the face of oncology in the country.

In the India of the 1940s, cancer was considered a deadly and incurable disease, resulting in almost certain death. 'The general public had not heard of such a disease, and in the classical Indian tradition classified it in the idea of *"karma vathigal"*, diseases destined by fate for which there could be no prevention and from which there could be no escape except through the gates of death,' wrote Krishnamurthi.[314] The idea of setting up a facility to cure people was thought to be throwing good money into a sinkhole. There was huge resistance, even within the medical community.

At the time, the only facility for cancer was the Tata Memorial in Mumbai. Yet, there was still no support for setting up another institute. Incensed, Dr Krishnamurthi gave a scathing address at the Hon. Medical Officers Conference on Cancer: 'There is enough wealth in our nation to perpetrate an evil and vicious caste of high priests; there is generosity enough to thrust memorials on men whose very lives were lived to demonstrate their emptiness, there is enough humanity to make a fetish and fashion of Ahimsa [an ancient Indian practice of non-violence, later adopted by Mahatma Gandhi], but there is neither money nor wealth nor generosity nor humanity to build a home for the poor sufferers of cancer. I think it is time we transferred a little of our Ahimsa from our books into our lives.'[315]

Dr Krishnamurthi began by setting up a cancer unit in the Government General Hospital, but this soon ran into difficulties. There was immense corruption and exploitation of patients, and pressure to admit influential patients ahead of others. Dr Shanta recounts an incident where Dr Krishnamurthi hit back at callous and ignorant government officials, during a visit by the health minister. The minister remarked that cancer affected only the old, so treatment was futile. An angry Dr Krishnamurthi responded, 'Sir, I speak from the statistics of our department and not from the statistics of others. My register shows quite a number of cancers in children, and cancers in adolescents. Pediatric cancer constitutes 8% of all cancers in government hospitals.'[316] He then produced the meticulously maintained register. The minister was furious and left in a huff.

Soon after, the cancer unit was closed, and all records confiscated. This was the last straw, which made Dr Reddy and Dr Krishnamurthi decide that it would be better to set up a separate cancer facility.

Now came Muthulakshmi's time to use all the contacts she had made over a lifetime in the public eye. And use them she did. She tried every minister, every prominent citizen and every powerful industrialist. She realised she needed a respected organisation to lend their name to the cause. The Women's Indian Association of Madras agreed.

When she approached the government of Tamil Nadu for land, a minister queried, 'Why a cancer hospital? People only die of cancer.'[317] After more pleading on her part, the government said that only one bit of land could be made available: 'a long narrow strip of 2 acres along the eastern bank of the Buckingham Canal in the district of Adyar'. The engineers found the land unsuitable, but the government said, 'take it or leave it'.[318]

The Cancer Institute (WIA)—also known as the Adyar Cancer Institute—still stands on that very same narrow, unsuitable strip of land, which apparently a number of visitors had criticised as poor planning and poor counsel. The foundation stone was laid on 10 October 1952 by Jawaharlal Nehru.

In the early years, Muthulakshmi travelled every month to Delhi to get funds to start the hospital. Initially, the hospital had only twelve beds and survived on borrowed equipment.

Dr Krishnamurthi took on the responsibility of running the institute in 1959, aided by the very young Dr Shanta. Its beginnings were spartan. Dr Shanta worked for three years on a voluntary basis, for a nominal salary of 200 rupees per month. Dr Shanta had been deeply moved by Nehru's stirring speeches urging citizens of newly independent India to work towards making the country self-reliant; she was inspired enough to work in an area completely unexplored at the time: oncology.

By 1960, there was recognition that children too suffered from cancer, and a paediatric ward was opened. Mortality was high, making for distressing experiences. 'In those days, we lost everybody,' recalls Dr Shanta. 'The children died. Their parents cried, and I cried with them. I am proud that today we have a 65 per cent improvement in paediatric cancer survival.'[319]

When the Emergency came in 1976, Indira Gandhi visited the hospital, and oddly took against it for reasons of her own. The doctors were suddenly evacuated and told that the hospital would affect the 'ecology' of Adyar. But Dr Krishnamurthi persevered. 'We will return,'[320] he said, quoting General McArthur. And they did, only a year later, when Indira Gandhi was defeated in the elections.

The Cancer Institute would go on to achieve many firsts, not just in India, but in Asia, competing with the best across the world. It would also pioneer medical oncology as a speciality, building knowledge from the ground up. As early as 1957, it would be the first centre in Asia to install a Cobalt 60 unit—a radiation treatment for cancer. It would be the first to install a paediatric oncology unit, the motto of which was 'They shall always have a tomorrow'. From those early twelve beds, it would grow to 450 beds.

'Dr Muthulakshmi always said, "No institute should be named after me",' said Dr Shanta.[321] Indeed, apart from a faded photograph of her in the institute, there is no mention of her name.

'Women In High Positions'

It is not hard to identify Muthulakshmi's legacy. The solid facade of the Adyar Cancer Institute, with its long lines of patients, the girls educated in the Avvai Home, the numerous social welfare schemes, the abolition of the devadasi system, and the winning of the vote for women are evidence enough. Add to this, her battle to bring women into public life, which was every bit as important.

In her later years, she would continue to be tirelessly active, despite declining eyesight due to glaucoma. 'We called her our Helen Keller,' says Dr Shanta.[322] Muthulakshmi became the first female alderman of the then Madras (now Chennai) Corporation and was awarded the Padma Bhushan in 1956.

When Muthulakshmi passed away in 1968, Indira Gandhi said on the radio, 'Were it not for women like Muthulakshmi and Dr Sarojini Naidu, we would not be occupying the high positions that we do today.'[323]

Perhaps Muthulakshmi's most profound legacy is the women she inspired to take the path less travelled. Dr Shanta died in January 2021, nearly ninety-four, but still in her position as chairman of the Adyar Cancer Institute. She lived in the same two humble rooms that she had always done, on the top floor of the old building of the institute, scattered with photographs, awards and books. After all these years of struggle, her passion for the institute still burned strongly, every bit as strongly as Muthulakshmi's.

'Looking back after 55 years, we had often wondered what made us go on under such hard conditions. It was probably the stubborn refusal to accept defeat, the faith that our patients had in us, the belief that having undertaken a mission, we have to continue, and follow the tenets of the Bhagavad Gita. Action is thy duty, fruit is not thy concern,' she wrote when Dr Krishnamurthi died.[324]

Action. Not accolades. Muthulakshmi would have approved.

CHAPTER SEVEN

The Surgeon General

Mary Poonen Lukose

'My father used to say, "My child, you have come to have certain advantages and privileges which other girls have not. Remember that you have responsibilities also."'

In May 2018, a curiously named man died, at the age of nearly one hundred. By any standards, Mikhail Savarimuthu had had a historic life, right from the beginning—he was Kerala's first C-section baby. The origin of his odd name is unclear. At the time he was born, in 1920, the Russian revolution had just swept the world's imagination, so he may have been named after the Bolshevik revolutionaries. The tiny rebel—who later became a soldier and then a clerk—came into the world with the help of one of our most interesting lady doctors, Mary Poonen Lukose.

Mary was a gynaecologist and obstetrician, who became not only the first female surgeon general in India, but also likely in the world. At least, there exist no reports of any other female surgeon generals at the time. To put that achievement in perspective, Mary was appointed in 1938. The first American woman surgeon general, Dr Antonia Novello, was appointed a full fifty-two years later, in 1990.

Mary owed her appointment to a visionary woman ruler: Sethu Lakshmi Bayi, the then ruler of Travancore, who pushed for women in every field: medicine, law and politics. Mary would be her durbar (royal household) physician, and shape Kerala's much-praised public health system. In 1924, she would also become the first woman legislator of India (Muthulakshmi Reddy is often credited as the first woman legislator on a technicality, but if you consider the princely state of Travancore to be a full-fledged state, then Mary was the first).

We know of Mary's life largely through her incomplete memoir that she began as a student, but sadly abandoned after her marriage.

Service To Your Sisters

'May in Ayemenem is a hot and brooding month. The days are long and humid. The river shrinks and black crows gorge on hot mangoes, in still dust green trees. Red bananas ripen. Jackfruits burst. Dissolute blue bottles hum vacuously in the fruity air...'[325]

These are the evocative first lines of Arundhati Roy's Booker Prize-winning novel, *The God of Small Things*. And it was in this languid village that Mary grew up.

The Syrian Christian community, to which Mary belonged, was a privileged and respected one, though not as privileged as some. At the top of the Travancore caste ladder were the Nambudiri Brahmins. The largest and most important section of society was the Nayars (or Nairs). But the Syrian Christians were on par with the Nayars in terms of status. They also had the advantage of being close to English missionaries, and thus close to 'English education, Malayalam printed books and a wide circle of connections.'[326] Indeed, unlike those from the historically oppressed castes, the Syrians 'walked where they pleased and carried only a minimum of pollution according to caste Hindus'. Despite their conversion to Christianity, they did not stop 'regarding lower caste Hindus as unclean.'[327]

Mary was an only child. Her father, Dr T.E. Poonen, was a doctor as well; he studied ophthalmology in Aberdeen University and was the first medical graduate in Travancore state. He would serve as the superintendent of the General Hospital in Thiruvananthapuram, and then go on to be the royal physician of Travancore. Mary's mother was constantly ill, so at the age of seven, Mary moved to Quilon, and was brought up entirely by her father.

This very unusual arrangement had far-reaching consequences. Like many of the lady doctors mentioned earlier, Mary was deeply influenced by her father, whose royal connections would help her greatly. Privileged they may have been, but T.E. Poonen would make sure that Mary was constantly aware of it. He always reminded her how lucky she was to be educated, when girls around her were being married off at thirteen, as was common amongst Syrian Christians. Therefore, he argued, she had responsibilities as well. 'The words he dinned into my ears time and time again were "service, service to your sisters". I must now admit quite frankly that at that early age these words meant very little to me for the simple reason that my experience of the ups and downs of life was so limited...' wrote Mary in her memoir.[328] But very soon, her father's lectures began to make sense to Mary. In 1909, she achieved one of her earliest firsts: she earned a BA from Madras University and became the first woman from Travancore to get a university degree. In those days, Malayali women were not allowed to get degrees in science, so she had to content herself with a degree in the arts.[329] But her father had already been making enquiries with universities in the United Kingdom, determined she should follow in his footsteps and get a British medical degree.

'The Land Of Ambition'

In 1909, the young Mary embarked on her voyage to the UK, having hurriedly learnt a bit of Latin from a Jesuit priest, which was a prerequisite for admission to British universities. Her voyage, on the Anchor

Line steamer service from Colombo, would take three whole weeks. Her father's princely connections would prove beneficial. She was looked after by the wife of the British resident in Travancore, Mrs Carr. The journey was a rough one, but Mary escaped seasickness. She writes, delightedly, of her 'first taste of a delicious pear eaten with cream' at a restaurant in Marseilles.[330]

Mary was awed by London. In her memoir, she calls her newly adopted country, 'The British Isles: The Land towards which All Ambition Turned'.[331]

It was a grandiose title, but it would prove true.

In October 1909, she began studying at the Royal Free Hospital, which was associated with the London School of Medicine. It was nineteen years since Rukhmabai had studied at the very same college. Mary had been granted admission with a degree in the arts, though the British women there had studied chemistry and physics. She was the only student from India. Photos from the time show her as a square-faced, strong-featured woman with a determined chin and wavy hair bobbed in the fashion of the time. Rather than wear a sari, she wore a long skirt with a high-necked blouse, helping her fit in with the British women students.

If it was difficult being the only Indian student at this time, her memoir doesn't reflect it. Her entries remain resolutely cheery and joyful, talking about her numerous travels in Britain and Scotland, her many friends, her trips to Selfridges and her sampling of the choicest Christmas pudding in Tottenham Court Road (she sent a sample to her father, as well). Her Kottayam connections helped her immensely. Her first Christmas was spent with the Bakers, a family that had set up a school for the education of women in Kottayam.

Mary wrote nothing about racial discrimination in her memoir. This was very much in keeping with her general no-nonsense attitude, and her distaste for whining. Having gone so far, she was clearly not going to moan. There is just one comical mention, when a five-year-old child, who had been told an 'Indian' was visiting, mistook her for a native American and remarked, 'But daddy, she has no feathers in her hair.'[332]

Many years later, in an interview with the Malayalam magazine *Vanitha*, Mary finally recalled an incident in London, where she stayed in a student hostel for young women. Every morning, when she walked onto the street, the neighbourhood children would gather around to shout 'Blackie, Blackie'. Once, they asked if she knew any English. Mary looked at her watch and replied with the time in a pukka British accent, causing utter confusion. 'Oh, she knows English, wonderful!' they shouted in disbelief.[333] Her response was typical of her cheery common sense.

Even as Mary entered university in 1909, London was experiencing an epic, monumental force: the suffragettes, so named for their commitment to suffrage for women, led by Emmeline Pankhurst. British women were still being denied the vote, even as other nations had enfranchised their women citizens.

In 1903, Pankhurst had started the Women's Social and Political Union (WSPU), which soon took to radical means. They chained themselves to railings, tried to storm parliament, jeered at politicians, set fire to empty buildings and even placed bombs in churches. When arrested, they went on hunger strikes, and were brutally force-fed. A woman named Emily Davison died when she ran in front of King George V's horse during the 1913 Epsom Derby.

The suffragettes' brave and pioneering campaign of civil disobedience influenced many, including Mahatma Gandhi. He visited London in 1909, the same year Mary arrived. 'The British women who have been demanding the franchise,' he wrote in his journal *Indian Opinion*, 'are putting up a wonderful show. They are not deterred by any kind of suffering. Every day a number of them keep standing the whole night near Parliament gate with the intention of handing in a petition to Mr Asquith [Herbert Asquith, the then British Prime Minister].

This is no ordinary courage. What great faith they must have! We can learn quite a few things and draw much inspiration from it.'[334] Gandhi would later distance himself from the violence of the suffragettes, but he remained an admirer.

Mary's memoir makes no mention of the suffragettes, but it is unlikely that she remained unaffected by the headlines of the time. She is reported to have met Sarojini Naidu at a public meeting and was 'bewitched by her oratorical prowess', though the date is unspecified. One imagines these astonishing events in London may have influenced her later, when Mary became involved in Travancore's efforts to bring in more women into the legislature, judiciary and administration.

Life At The LSM

Mary writes very little about her course at the LSM, but we know some details from the accounts of other students who were her contemporaries. One such person whose records survive, was Ethel Brand, who attended the institute about eight years before Mary.

In 1901, when Ethel entered the school, records show that the fees were 125 pounds in all, about 10,000 pounds now. The course could take over five years, and by some estimates, the cost of accommodation and examination fees could be over 1,000 pounds.[335]

How did Mary pay for it? Records show that she received a scholarship from the then maharaja of Travancore, Sree Moolam Thirunal, who her father served as physician. Mary was given 200 pounds per year, on the condition that she return to Travancore and serve the government for ten years, as a sort of bond. She was also required to furnish a security of immovable property valued at 15,000 rupees.[336] She was thus immensely lucky to receive this kind of support, and to be privileged enough to have property at her disposal.

Mary does not write of the prejudice against women medical students, but again, accounts of the time show us that they continued to be treated with disdain by the male fraternity. In 1911, when Mary was about halfway through her course, Marie Curie won the Nobel Prize for chemistry for the second time. Yet, as a doctor and medical historian points out, regardless of Curie's two wins, it was also the year in which the female students of the Royal Free Hospital had to listen to an infuriating address by Sir Henry Butlin, president of the Royal College of Surgeons, in which he questioned the ability of women to do medical research. Butlin's condescending speech ended thus, 'I have no doubt I shall be asked whether I believe that women will be found competent for research, whether they have the breadth of mind necessary for such work, and whether they will ever be able to do more than carry out researches that have been designed for them. Indeed I do not know. But I should certainly like to see them try.'[337]

Even decades later, the situation remained unchanged. When Sir Robert Hutchison, president of the Royal College of Physicians, addressed the students and graduates of the Royal Free in 1941, he began with some slight praise, and then went on to share his real opinion. 'When a woman doctor is bad she's horrid—even horrider than a bad man doctor,' he said. He also advised women doctors not to be 'too high and mighty' when applying for jobs; and at interviews, 'if you paint your nails, you are infallibly and quite rightly damned'. At work, 'women are more apt to let their work get on top of them', 'general practice is hard work and many women cannot stand the strain of it' and 'medical women make excellent wives, while their qualification is always a second string to their bow.'[338]

Hutchison's views were shared by most medical men of the time.

British Women In 1910: Quiet Desperation

What was life like for women in early 20th century England with no national health service, a social welfare system or modern household appliances? The answer was: mostly bleak. Women, of course, did not have the vote yet. They were also denied higher education, and expected to be full-time wives and mothers. Working-class girls of course had it even worse, learning little in school beyond domestic subjects such as cookery, laundry and childcare. This meagre education condemned them to poorly paid jobs, usually in domestic service or factories. 'The lowest paid was the maid-of-all-work or general servant, earning 12 to 18 pounds a year, plus board and lodging. Other single working-class women might earn 13 shillings a week (65p) in the non-textile industries, but even that was not enough for a fully independent existence.'[339]

Marriage thus became the only way out for most working-class women. But that often entailed grinding poverty, overcrowded slum housing and gruelling physical labour. Most working-class wives did not know of birth control, and had to manage growing families on a pound a week. Even when pregnant, a wife might live on bread and jam. Often, the baby died young. Women often tried dangerous methods to end a pregnancy—knitting needles, bottles of gin, hot baths, throwing themselves down the stairs.

There was no heating at the time, except for open fires, which had to be constantly fed with coal. Clothes had to be washed by hand in a tub. Not surprisingly, the life expectancy for women was only fifty-five, in contrast with around eighty-two as of 2010.[340]

These then were the patients that Mary saw, the poorest of the poor, made wretched by hard work, constant child-bearing and the lack of proper medical care. While working at Dublin's Rotunda Hospital in 1914, Mary helped deliver babies in 'squalid backstreets' and slum quarters, where entire families shared one room. When women were brought to bed, husbands would often be out at work, she wrote. 'I distinctly remember one instance where, while I was attending on the woman, her husband was fast asleep in another corner of the room, so dead-tired from this night's toil that he did not even hear the first cry of a newborn, and knew of the arrival of a son only when I woke him up by shaking his shoulder.'[341]

Often, the medical students had to do everything from boiling water to taking care of the many little children in the house. 'When there were no other means in sight, we students bore the expenses ourselves for providing some snacks for the children.'[342]

Mary wrote of her disappointment at not having enough exposure to the treating of infectious diseases like cholera, typhoid, smallpox and chickenpox in London. On one occasion, the students rushed to see a supposed case of typhoid, but it turned out to be a false alarm. But the intrepid doctor travelled all over the UK to observe the effects of different conditions, including those affecting the mind. 'Mental cases not far advanced in illnesses were allowed to be at large within the enclosed area, and their erratic movements and vacant stares often put us on our guard,' she wrote.[343]

Then, in 1914, the war came. Mary was in Northampton. She decided to travel to the Rotunda Hospital, where she intended to get more experience in gynaecology. On the way, she encountered war refugees from the continent. 'Men and women—young and old—and children of all ages were there, stripped of all their possessions, many among them bereft of their near and dear ones. I could see nothing but misery, all round lamentations, weeping and wailing.' Mary spent the night in a hotel chair, because there were no beds available.[344] Eventually, she arrived in Dublin. The city was fairly insulated from the war, and the Rotunda was a shelter for Mary. It was here that she discovered her true calling: aiding women to give birth safely. She would spend two years there, and handle nearly three hundred cases.

Amongst her gurus was Dr E.H. Tweedy, a much-respected Irish gynaecologist. Mary's first operation was with his supervision and encouragement. Dr Tweedy was operating in the gallery, when he suddenly called Mary down. Thinking she was called upon to assist with instruments, she went down unsuspectingly. Dr Tweedy then handed her the knife and asked her to 'carry on'. Mary was terrified.

'In a flurry of excitement, I stood transfixed with my eyes riveted on the doctor. Before I could collect myself, pat came the admonition: "What are you staring at me for? Carry on—don't you see I am here?"

I was overwhelmed with a consciousness of diffidence and timidity.'
Mary's hands were trembling, but she had no choice but to do as asked.
It was a simple hysterectomy, and it went off perfectly. From then on,
she was allowed to perform numerous operations.[345]

Mary graduated in October 1915 with an MBBS, and was awarded
five guineas by none other than Mary Scharlieb. With it, she bought a
gold watch and bracelet, which became family heirlooms. As the war
wore on, male doctors were overstretched, so women were brought in.
Mary worked for three gruelling months in a military hospital, helping
the wounded.

Return To Mayvil

Mary had many professional opportunities in the UK, but in March
1916, her beloved father died at the age of only fifty-seven. Mary was
distraught. Her father had guided her every step of the way. Mary now
had to make her own decisions. Should she leave the UK, where positions for medical women were growing, and return to India, where her
future was uncertain? Her many friends came to her aid.

Dr Scharlieb told her about the vacancy for a lady doctor in the
medical department of Travancore state. The post had always been occupied by a British doctor and Mary would be the first Indian woman to
be considered. Before she could accept, she was offered an even greater
honour. The maharaja of Travancore gave her the post of senior surgeon
in charge of the Women and Children's Hospital, Trivandrum. He also
sent her 1,000 rupees—a huge sum of money at the time.

Mary returned to India after a long and perilous sea voyage.
On board her ship was 'an important person carrying a crucial war
message'. The ship was camouflaged, as was the usual practice then.
The Germans wanted to bring her ship down, but they torpedoed and
sank another ship by mistake, off the straits of Messina. Mary's ship
narrowly escaped destruction.

On her return to Travancore, a desolate Mary found her childhood home, Mayvil, empty and deserted. All her father's possessions had been removed and sold. Later, Mary would tell her daughter in law, Aley Lukose, 'I went to England like a princess and came back like an orphan.'[346]

Travancore's Massive Health Campaign

But Mary had no time to brood or grieve for her father. She was quickly drafted into the state of Travancore's mammoth efforts to improve maternal health. Sree Moolam Thirunal was keen to improve the healthcare of women and girls, but had been blocked at every turn by the social attitudes of the time.

In 1916, Trivandrum (now Thiruvananthapuram)—the capital of Travancore state—was changing from a sleepy, small city to a centre of education and culture. Under the reign of Maharaja Swathi Thirunal, about a century earlier, the first English school (now the University College), an observatory, a general hospital and the Oriental Research Institute and Manuscripts Library had all been set up. Moolam Thirunal set up several more colleges, including the Sanskrit College, Law College and the Ayurveda College.

Still, with all this education, women were reluctant to go to hospitals. Mary came to a hospital which had ninety-one beds, but only twenty patients. In 1916, only 150 cases were treated in the entire hospital. Mary explained why: 'The feeling had somehow gained ground that hospitals were like poor homes, meant for the poor, the uncared, the abandoned and that confinement of a patient to a hospital, was for the patient, nothing less than sure death. The only women who resorted to hospital treatment in times of illness and for confinement and delivery were those in the lowest strata of society.'[347]

Most often, she would receive patients who had been mistreated by midwives, or quacks, and were in the last stages of their lives. 'The maternity cases brought to hospital were almost always advanced septic cases... In most cases nothing could be done by the doctors in hospital to save either the mother or child or both. It was this circumstance that gave currency to the unfortunate impression even in educated and forward circles that patients admitted to hospitals, as a rule, succumbed to their maladies.'[348]

Marriage: 'I Have Been Waiting For You'

By the time Mary returned to Mayvil in 1916, she was thirty years old, more than twice the usual age for a bride. Mary had been too busy with her career to think of marriage, but now that Mayvil lay empty, her thoughts began to turn to it.

It is in 1917 that her memoir sadly ends. Whatever we know of her after that is from the accounts of her relatives, letters and newspaper articles. Like many women, perhaps Mary was simply too busy with work, marriage, children and running a house to maintain a diary.

She would make a very unconventional marriage, in keeping with her unconventional life. Her future husband, Kannukuzhiyil Kuruvilla Lukose, was a lawyer. Scandalously for the time, he was also younger than her. He would eventually become a judge of the Travancore High Court, and be called 'Judgie' for short. Pictures of Judgie show a man with large, expressive eyes and curly hair, and a strong resemblance to Charlie Chaplin. Judgie would prove to have a similar sense of humour. When Mary asked Judgie why he had not married earlier, he responded blithely, 'I have been waiting for you.'[349]

Judgie and Mary married in 1917, and settled down contentedly in Mayvil, on the road now known as Poonen Road after her father, where she would live for the rest of her life. Judgie was not intimidated by his brilliant wife's long list of accomplishments. 'Every year, they had to go to the Palace on the Maharajah's birthday, and would each be presented with a traditional *kavani* (shawl),' wrote Mary's daughter-in-law, Aley Lukose. 'The width of the gold border of the kavani depended on the recipient's rank or station. Her kavani had a four-inch border, while her husband's was three inches wide.'[350]

Mary would go on to have two children in quick succession: Grace Lukose, born in 1918, and K.P. Lukose, born in 1920. Grace would go on to become a doctor, studying in the UK just as her mother did. K.P. would study at Balliol College in Oxford, and go on to become the permanent representative of India to the UN and later, the Indian ambassador to Bulgaria.

Then, as now, women who worked outside the home were still supposed to prioritise their family and house. In 1966, a public meeting with a gathering of distinguished guests was held to celebrate Mary's eightieth birthday. K.P. Lukose would send a message to be read out which he described as the 'thoughts as the progeny of a mother who during the most impressionable years of my life, was to an uncommon extent occupied in duties and activities outside the home'. Still, he took pains to emphasise, her 'obligation' as a wife and mother remained central to her. 'The diet of her husband, the clothing of the children, illness in the family, in all these it was her provisioning and supervising that ensured that nothing lacked. Not a detail of our performance at school slipped her notice.'[351]

Other guests also repeated that she had never neglected her family duties. 'She has been an ideal mother, and ideal wife and an ideal grandmother,' said K.P.S. Menon, India's first foreign secretary, in his speech at the same occasion. The message was that women could excel outside the home, provided they fulfilled their primary duties at home. If Mary resented this double burden, she did not mention it anywhere.

Friends In Need

Mary's son also noted the multicultural nature of the household. Indeed, over the course of her life, Mary made a huge number of friends, not just amongst the Syrian Christians, but also amongst the Nair community, the British community and various others.

Of these many friends, the most unusual and mercurial was certainly Dr Theodore Howard Somervell, a British surgeon who spent nearly forty years working in India. Like most Western doctors in India at that time, he was a missionary. Dr Somervell was not just a doctor—he was also a world-class mountaineer and member of two Everest expeditions, an Olympic gold medallist and a painter.

One time, Mary was waiting for Somervell in front of his room, when he suddenly appeared in another room, to which there was no other entrance than the one she could see. Apparently, Somervell, then planning another Everest expedition, had scaled the wall of the hospital and climbed up a palm tree to enter the room.[352]

Somervell was a member of the ill-fated 1924 Everest expedition, where the mountaineers George Mallory and Andrew Irvine disappeared. Somervell barely escaped with his life, ascending to 8,500 metres, less than a kilometre from the summit, before he was forced to turn back because of a very sore throat. His record would not be officially beaten until Edmund Hillary and Tenzing Norgay climbed Everest in 1952 (though there has always been speculation that Mallory and Irvine also conquered Everest).[353]

So modest was Somervell that even his own family did not realise he had won an Olympic gold medal, until they went through his belongings after his death. The medal was one of twenty-one awarded to mountaineers on the 1922 Everest expedition, the first full expedition, when mountaineering was considered an Olympic sport.[354]

Somervell began working in India at the Neyyoor Hospital in 1923. Then a part of the state of Travancore, it is now in the Kanyakumari district of Tamil Nadu. As Mary ceased writing her memoir in 1916, we have no accounts of what she found when she arrived in Travancore. But Dr Somervell's detailed memoir, *Knife and Life in India: Being the Story of a Surgical Missionary at Neyyoor, Travancore*, paints a vivid picture of medical life a few years later in 1920s Travancore, and thus fills the gap.

Somervell wrote passionately about how difficult—often impossible—it was to persuade Indians to come to the hospital, especially women. Though the women of Travancore did better than women in many parts of India, they still led incredibly secluded lives and were reluctant to seek medical help until they were almost dying.

Somervell's innovative tactics to win the confidence of the residents make for fascinating reading. To allay their fears of surgery, Somervell introduced an open gallery system, where relatives and friends of the patient could watch the operation. 'Some years ago I learned that many patients believed that a surgical operation meant "making a hole in the stomach and letting a devil out" the devil being responsible for the disease. We wish to show to such people that an operation is a carefully conducted and rational procedure, and in many cases we can show them the actual disease, for instance the scar of an ulcer in the stomach, or the mass of a malignant growth.'[355]

Somervell also wrote about how incredibly difficult it was to persuade women to break through their seclusion and be seen by male doctors. He was once asked by a highly educated and well-placed Indian man to see his wife. When he got there, he found another Indian doctor there, who told him he had been treating the patient for years, but had never been allowed to be in the same room as her. 'One day they tied a string to her wrist and asked me to hold the other end of it, in the next room, and by that means to feel her pulse. That is the nearest approach to a clinical examination that I have ever been permitted to make.'[356]

Elsewhere, Somervell wrote a heartfelt account of the many quacks in Travancore, most of them native healers or 'vaidyans'. Like Mary, he too found that most residents would try the quacks first, who promised quick cures, then the homeopath, and only when they were desperate would they come to doctors. In one tragic case, he met a young girl who had had typhoid and gone to the village vaidyan. The vaidyan believed that the devil responsible for typhoid fever lived in her eyes and so had put green chilli paste in her eyes. The girl was in tremendous pain for several days, and when the paste was finally removed, it was found that both her eyes were destroyed. The patient had recovered from typhoid, but her eyes would never recover.

Often, the native healers would administer drugs in excess, sometimes of 'over fifty times the lethal dose'. Somervell's own junior doctor contracted leprosy, and despite his warnings, went to a vaidyan. He died in agony, of phosphorus and mercury poisoning, and just managed to say, '*Salaam. Naan pogiren.*' Which means 'Goodbye, I am gone.' He was cured of leprosy, but killed by the drug overdose.[357]

This was the incredibly difficult setting in which Mary had to make her way, handicapped by being a woman, an Indian and also a Syrian Christian. Somervell helped her out in many instances. In one case, Mary performed a caesarean surgery to save a pregnant woman, when it was clear that the baby could not be saved. The relatives of the woman sued her for not saving the baby. Dr Somervell cited medical jurisprudence to argue that caesarean operations were recommended in cases where the mother's life was at stake. Mary won the case.

Somervell would have a deep influence on Mary, but there was another who would have an even greater influence.

The Queen And I

In 1916, Mary met a woman who would change her life in every way. Sethu Lakshmi Bayi, who would later become the senior maharani (senior queen) of Travancore, was as much an oddity as Mary was.

The royal family of Travancore was a curious beast in the otherwise patriarchal society of India. In the matrilineal tradition of Kerala, as historian and author Manu Pillai puts it, 'A family did not take after the patriarchal model of man, wife and their children. Instead, it consisted to put it simplistically, of man, sister and her children. The crown passed not from father to son, but from maternal uncle to nephew, and the Rani was never the maharajah's wife, but his sister or niece or great-niece.'[358]

Thus, the reigning king at any time would not have inherited from his father, but from his mother and her brother, if any. In fact, the sons of the maharajas and the husbands of the ranis had no power or status at all. 'In the matrilineal system, it did not matter who your father was, as much as who your mother and uncle were.'[359]

In this matrilineal society, girls were sought after, so that they could produce heirs. If there were no male heirs, girls were eligible to inherit the throne.

Sethu Lakshmi Bayi and her cousin Sethu Parvati Bayi were adopted into the royal family in 1900, to serve as 'backups' for the princes. They were both granddaughters of the painter Raja Ravi Varma.

As prospective heirs, both princesses were brought up in splendour and luxury, but also with rigorous etiquette and protocol. Sethu Lakshmi Bayi, the older by a year, was called 'the Senior Rani', and Sethu Parvati Bayi, 'the Junior Rani'.

Shut away in the fabulous Sundara Vilasam Palace in Trivandrum, the princesses lead luxurious but lonely lives. They were allowed no playmates outside of the royal family, and were educated by private tutors in Malayalam, Sanskrit and English. They also learnt history, arithmetic, music, painting and other skills expected of princesses.

When she was ten, Sethu Lakshmi Bayi was married to Rama Varma, a noble from a related house. Sethu Parvati Bayi was also married to another member of the nobility. Mary became the personal physician of the two ranis in 1916, replacing a British physician.

A 'race' ensued between the Senior and Junior ranis to bear heirs to the throne. It was a race that the Junior Rani won comprehensively. She had three children by 1922, including two male successors to the throne. Mary was the physician for these births, a huge responsibility.

Meanwhile, Sethu Lakshmi Bayi had suffered a series of painful miscarriages and one traumatic stillbirth of a boy at eight months, but had no children. In royal circles, she began to be called 'barren' and 'cursed', making her feel even more isolated and lonely.

But in 1923, when Sethu Lakshmi Bayi was twenty-eight and had been married for over seventeen years, the unexpected happened. The Senior Rani began feeling tired and nauseous, and was found to be pregnant. Given her history, she was incredibly nervous. The atmosphere was fraught. Mary found herself caretaker to an intensely wanted and needed baby, and also the first Indian woman to take on such a massive responsibility. She rose to the occasion.

Immense care was taken, but the baby arrived a month early, and the Senior Rani went into an eclamptic fit. It was safe, but was underweight, and the Senior Rani was severely ill. Mary insisted that the nursery was kept scrupulously clean, and the baby wrapped in several layers of cotton and flannel sheets to stay warm. The baby was kept indoors for six months, until it began thriving. The tiny scrap of a thing was given a name almost longer than she was: Her Highness Uthram Thirunal Lalithamba Bayi Tampuran, the second princess of Travancore. And with this, Mary earned the undying gratitude of the Senior Rani.

The Senior Rani would have barely enough time to enjoy motherhood before a crisis hit. In August 1924, Sree Moolam Thirunal, the maharaja of Travancore and Mary's father figure, died. The heir to the throne was the Junior Rani's twelve-year-old son, Chitira Thirunal, who was too young to be king. According to custom, the Senior Rani was anointed regent, until he would come of age. She was only twenty-nine years old. Suddenly, she found herself the de facto ruler of Travancore, an unexpected development for a shy and retiring woman who had never thought to find herself in this position. Nevertheless, she would go on to shape Travancore and change its culture and institutions forever. Her radical reforms would make Malayali women the envy of India.

The Pioneering Women Of Kerala

Sethu Lakshmi Bayi's views on the role of women were conservative in some aspects and broadminded in others. In many ways, she was a true Victorian puritan, and the model of wifely devotion, just as Queen Victoria was. She would go on to abolish the traditional matrilineal system and encourage patriarchal households. She insisted on her husband being included in all state functions, contrary to the prevailing custom. Thus far, the husband of the rani had been insignificant. Now, he was allowed to ride with her in her carriage and sit in her presence, shocking the people of Travancore.

However, as historians have pointed out, 'The cultural conservatism of the Maharani did not mean that she desired women to remain at home and withhold from participation in private life.'[360] For instance, in the mid-1920s, 'much excitement was aroused in Trivandrum when it was announced that all girls who went to college in the state would automatically be rewarded with an invitation to join their queen at her palace for tea.'[361]

The maharani would begin a massive campaign to encourage women to participate in the affairs of state, and the first of these was Mary.

Soon after the Senior Rani's succession as regent, Mary was appointed as the head of the medical department of Travancore. She was also nominated as a member of the Travancore Legislative Council, which made her India's first female legislator.

By now, Mary had become a mainstay of the royal family. In 1926, Sethu Lakshmi Bayi was expecting her second child. With the benefit of hindsight, Mary wrote a brisk letter asking for sheds to be prepared at Satelmond Palace, one for the surgeon—herself—two for another doctor and the nurses, and a tent for the officers of state. She also asked for the following items in a quaint letter:

One small cot for the baby
12 Pears soaps for the baby and 12 Vinolia Otto Toilet
soaps for the mother
4 long pillows with 4 covers for each
Six yards of silk and one roll silk ribbon for the baby's
clothing.[362]

At the time, Vinolia Otto was considered a most superior soap. It was the soap supplied to the first-class passengers on the *Titanic*.

The luxuriously wrapped and powdered baby would turn out to be a second girl, Her Highness Karthika Thirunal Indira Bayi.

In 1938, Mary would be appointed surgeon general of Travancore, likely the first woman surgeon general in the world. As surgeon general, she would be in charge of the health programme for the whole state. There were numerous obstacles. To begin with, white people were usually preferred for this post. 'There was a mania for white skin,' wrote Dr C.O. Karunakaran, the founder of the Government Medical College in Trivandrum.[363] Also, Mary was competing with a renowned surgeon, Raman Thampi. It took her many years to over-come these prejudices, and she was eventually appointed only when she was thought sufficiently experienced. The progress of the state under the control of the Rani and Mary in tandem was remarkable. In 1920, there were sixty state-run medical institutions. By 1946, this had grown to a hundred and forty. Thanks to the matrilineal system, girl children in Kerala had always been more educated than their coun-terparts in the rest of India. But due to the Rani's push for female education, more and more girls were educated. As historian Robin Jeffrey pointed out, 'When Dr Poonen Lukose first became a durbar physician in 1924, 15 percent of Travancore women were literate, more than seven times the all-Indian proportion. When she retired in 1942, close to half of all girls between the ages of 5 and 15 were at school, and female literacy in Travancore reached 36 per cent.'[364] An amazing achievement by any standards.

Battling It Out In The Legislative Council

A glance at the minutes of the Travancore Legislative Assembly proceedings show Mary fighting a lonely battle, often being ridiculed by male legislators who had no respect for her medical expertise. As Somervell had pointed out, there was a deep distrust of Western science and modern medicine. It made no difference that she was the physician of the royal family, and later, the surgeon general. From the proceedings, it is clear that to many of them, she was just a silly woman, unworthy of respect.

Mary was always calm and logical, despite attempts by male legislators to rattle her. Often, she remonstrated gently, 'I did not say that', or clarified her intention not to insult. Yet she stuck to her guns, always staunch in the cause of science and modern medicine. She painstakingly brought various motions to establish dispensaries, train nurses, introduce vaccination programmes, improve hygiene, eliminate rats and generally do the thankless work of building a health system from ground up. This was not a glamorous role, and Mary was impeded at every turn by those who did not believe in modern medicine.

Her first real battle was the fight for compulsory vaccination. In 1925, M.M. Madhava Varier, a legislator, attempted to move a resolution calling for vaccination in Travancore to be made optional. He wanted 'conscientious objectors' to vaccination to be allowed to forego it.

At the time, Mary and Sethu Lakshmi Bayi had worked long and hard to ensure that vaccinations were compulsory, and children could not be admitted to schools without them. Varier called vaccinations 'medical barbarism' and tried to present evidence that patients who were vaccinated still got smallpox. Indeed, he argued that the vaccination was more dangerous than smallpox. There followed a heated debate, in which male legislators argued about the efficacy of vaccines and the danger of introducing lymph into the system. Predictably, none of them were doctors, but that did not stop them. Supporting Varier was a well-known homeopath called M.N. Pillai. 'There is no reason why vaccines should be introduced into the human system,' he stated confidently. 'The lymph that is introduced creates a disease similar to smallpox.'[365]

Mary let the men argue for a while. Then she stepped in, firmly. 'I strongly oppose the resolution,' she said, and proceeded to explain why. Way before the concept of herd immunity and the damage caused by 'conscientious objectors' was widely known, Mary understood the ramifications. She tried to explain as best she could. Smallpox, she explained, is a disease spread by air, to a distance of at least half a mile. In crowded cities like Travancore, isolation of the patient was impossible, and often resisted, making vaccination the only option. 'Petty inconveniences and even risks have to be encountered by individuals for the sake of the greater good of the community as a whole,' she said. In saying this unapologetically, Mary was explaining the main principle underlying all public health: that of public cooperation. 'If you do not mind getting infected with smallpox, the matter does not end there. You are infecting other people who are not vaccinated.'[366]

Mary went on to cite irrefutable statistics showing that compulsory vaccination had reduced mortality rates in smallpox. She agreed that there were cases where vaccination caused inflammation, but argued that instead of making them voluntary, the quality and method of vaccinations should be improved. Eventually, Mary made a plea. 'We have a great deal of uphill work before us. The public needs to be handled tactfully. Much propaganda work has to be done.' Her cool logic and swift refutations to everything carried the day. Varier, perhaps convinced, withdrew the motion.

Then in 1928, her old foe, the homeopathic doctor M.N. Pillai, traded blows with her once again. As a qualified doctor, Mary was sceptical of homeopathy, but she had to tread cautiously because she was surrounded by its supporters. At the time, allopathy was still regarded with great suspicion, and homeopathy—with its fast-acting and cheap remedies—was highly respected.

Pillai proposed that the government introduce grants to support 'qualified' homeopathic practitioners. Mary was clearly aghast at scarce funds being used to prop up homeopathy, when people were still dying due to a lack of doctors. She tried to be diplomatic, refraining from denouncing homeopathy. Instead, she argued that there were very few qualified practitioners, and that therefore the government should not support the proposition. She pointed out that the majority of homeopathy practitioners in Travancore 'had not the slightest knowledge of anatomy, pathology or physiology.'[367]

There was instant outrage from the assembly. An incensed Pillai and his coterie of homeopathy fans began attacking allopathy in general and Mary in particular. 'There is this inherent hatred of allopathic doctors towards homeopathy from the very beginning,' said Pillai. His supporters alleged that allopaths were only in medicine to make money and prescribe unnecessary drugs. 'Give the people a chance to escape the drugging system,' yelled his supporter G. Raman Menon. Another supporter was the journalist K.C. Mammen Mappillai, the founder of the Malayala Manorama group of publications. Mappillai argued that there were not enough qualified medical doctors, and that the harmless resolution could help the poor get access to care. Another legislator, Dr A.K. Pillai, argued, incredibly, that the multiplying number of doctors, whether allopathic or homeopathic, was becoming a 'menace to society'. 'Too many cooks spoil the dish, so also, many doctors spoil the life of many people,' he said. Instead, he suggested, government aid should be reduced so 'people exist freely and peacefully without any embarrassment from doctors.'[368]

This ludicrous exchange sums up the deep suspicion of doctors in the Travancore of the time. It is to Mary's credit that she remained calm and rational in the face of these attacks. 'Most of the members who spoke said that homeopathy is convenient and cheap and useful in the treatment of children. It is no doubt convenient and cheap, but these considerations should not be taken into account. I am not convinced it is as efficacious as allopathy,' explained Mary, with all her experience behind her.[369] But it was not rationality's day. The supporters of homeopathy won, and the Kerala government decided to give grants to homeopathic practitioners. Homeopathy become popular, proceeding side by side with allopathy; it was subsequently encouraged further by chief minister E.M.S. Namboodiripad.

Even more than twelve years after she was appointed surgeon general, male legislators continued to behave patronisingly towards Mary. But by then, awarded the title of Vaidyasastrakusala (meaning, expert in the medical sciences) by the Travancore royals, she was quick to give as good as she got. In 1940, an MLA, Kochikal Balakrishna Thampi, criticised her treatment of a local resident on a hospital committee. 'Without meaning any offence,' said Thampi snidely, intending of course to give every offence, 'I would say that we must have as Surgeon General, a person with more Indian manners.' Clearly, there was some resentment with regard to Mary's foreign education and experience.

Mary did not let the statement slide. 'I must object to that remark, I am thoroughly Indian. It is true that I understand fairly well the customs and manners of Europeans, and I have travelled in European countries also. But I am equally proud to say I am an Indian to the very core and I understand Indian manners very well.'[370]

Mary had learnt to stand up for herself, and her demeanour served as a model for many educated Malayali women who had to deal with mansplaining, prejudice and condescension from men.

Loss And Sorrow

Mary would retire from service in 1942, at age fifty six. She would spend her later years with her three grandchildren, the children of her diplomat son K.P. Lukose, who fondly remembered her as 'Oma', the German word for grandmother. The children had adopted it when K.P. Lukose was posted in Bonn.

As K.P. Lukose and his wife Aley travelled the world, the grandchildren would spend time with their devoted Oma. Mary would feed them, tell them stories, slip them money and teach them how to drive. Every grandchild was also taken to meet the royal family at Kowdiar Palace.

Kuruvilla Lukose, her grandson, recalled a time when he and his cousin stole a bottle of brandy from Oma's cupboard. She was in her eighties then. 'We swigged by turn, making sure we did not empty the bottle completely. We were drinking [it] neat and felt the fire!' The next day, the two teenagers realised Oma had replaced the contents of the bottle with soya sauce.[371]

In her later years, Mary would also be the president of the Trivandrum YWCA, out of gratitude for the help they had rendered her in the UK.

Mary was to suffer a series of terrible losses in her old age. Both her children would die before her. Her much loved and brilliant daughter Grace had gone on to become an assistant professor in the Lady Hardinge Medical College in New Delhi by 1947. She would die prematurely in 1954—at only thirty-five—after a freak electrical accident in the UK.

K.P. Lukose, to whom Mary wrote every single week and sent a fruitcake every year to his various postings, died of a heart attack in 1975, aged fifty-four. Only a year later, Mary would pass away, at the age of ninety.

Her work to build Kerala's formidable public healthcare system would be remembered and inspire succeeding generations of healthcare professionals. During her tenure in government, she had not always got her due—especially from men—and faced much ridicule for her devotion to modern medicine. But her efforts paid off in the years to come. Kerala's robust public health system would grow in strength, and demonstrate amazing efficiency in combating the Nipah virus, the coronavirus pandemic and a host of other diseases. This was largely due to the foundations laid by Mary, and other rationalists like her.

As recently as 2018, Kerala's finance minister T.M. Thomas Isaac would mention her in his budget speech. 'Mary Poonen Lukose was one of the extraordinary talents who influenced the growth of the healthcare system in Kerala,' Isaac said, while praising the network of institutions she painstakingly built from scratch. 'The average lifespan that stood at 45—even at the time of the state formation—rose to 76.' The minister also warned of anti-vaxxers, whom Mary had fought so hard against. 'In this context, we should seriously view the organised opposition to vaccination and modern medicine that arise from certain corners, and not forget our past experience.'[372]

Epilogue

'I had even then set my heart upon something high and I wanted to be a different woman from the common lot.'
— Muthulakshmi Reddy

Six lady doctors from every corner of India. What did they have in common, and what impact did they have?

The lady doctors shared one thing: the encouragement of supportive men. In the case of Haimabati, Rukhmabai, Muthulakshmi and Mary, their fathers defied society to educate them. In the case of Anandibai and Kadambini, their husbands did.

This is not intended to detract from their achievements. It was a time when women found it hard to make it in a man's world without a man's support. And if the lady doctors received initial help that many other women did not, it is also true that they rapidly outgrew that need. The fathers died, the husbands stayed in India and yet the women went on to study overseas and work on their own.

If men aided them, it is also true that other men impeded them. The many instances where women students were bullied by their male counterparts and gave up their medals to them were forgiven by the lady doctors, but they should not be forgotten by us.

Another common feature was that all the women, except Rukhmabai and in part Muthulakshmi, were upper caste. Caste privilege certainly helped them up the ladder. It is worth noting that

Rukhmabai encountered more abuse and hatred than any of the other women, with entire newspapers devoted to vilifying her. Still, even the upper-caste women did not have a smooth ride. Haimabati's upper-class origins did not save her from harassment in the workplace. Mary's influential family could not prevent her being attacked as an 'outsider' in the legislature by resentful men.

These women had no role models to emulate or follow. There were precious few women in public life for them to idolise. It is notable that two of the lady doctors—Muthulakshmi and Mary—mentioned being inspired by Sarojini Naidu. Pandita Ramabai, though she never attained her dream of becoming a doctor, also served as a mentor of sorts to Rukhmabai.

Kadambini, with her eight children, made working motherhood acceptable, even aspirational. Haimabati, following closely behind, deftly managed her family and her job. This also had an unintentional consequence. Women like Kadambini and Mary were often praised for being good mothers and wives first, and good doctors next. Motherhood continued to be idolised, and defenders of Indian women doctors would argue that women made good doctors because selflessness came naturally to them. This was exactly what the early pioneers had argued against: the fetishisation of women doctors. Again, the trailblazing Rukhmabai was the only one who did not stay married, and still managed to build a reputation.

The impact of the lady doctors on medical education was huge. For one, they forced conservative colleges to throw open their doors to women, and indeed, take pride in women students. Kadambini's success left the Calcutta Medical College with no option but to allow women students. Overseas education, so unheard of for women in the time of Anandibai, became more acceptable. In 1912, the Government of India sanctioned a special scholarship for postgraduate education for women, which had so far been reserved for men. Jerusha Jhirad, a Jewish medical student from India's tiny Bene Israeli community, became the first woman to be awarded the scholarship. Jhirad already had a degree in medicine from Grant Medical College, and went on to study at the London School of Medicine, following in the path of Rukhmabai and earning an MD in obstetrics and gynaecology. Jhirad returned to India to become superintendent at the Madame Cama Hospital.

Bombay, and the Grant Medical College in particular, became a centre for women doctors. By 1913, sixty-six women, including Europeans, Eurasians, Parsis, Indian Christians, Hindus and Jews, had secured the Licentiate of Medicine and Surgery (LMS) degrees from the college. It is impossible to list all the women who helped make the Bombay Presidency a leader in healthcare, but along with Jhirad, Rani Rajwade, Dosibai Dadabhoy and Malini Sukthankar played significant roles in public health and planning.

The lady doctors also helped destroy colonial prejudice and dismantle the structure of 'zenana medicine', where only British women doctors were considered worthy of leading. Kadambini's battle against the Dufferin Fund made people take Indian women doctors more seriously. Haimabati and other humble VLMSs underlined the importance of the Indian lady doctor in rural areas.

Consequently, medical associations were set up to train more women doctors: the Association of Medical Women of India in 1907, and the Women's Medical Service in 1909. Rukhmabai was made a member of the AMWI in 1912, and the WMS too. To begin with, these organisations were dominated by British women. But by 1949, thanks to the tireless demands of Indian women doctors such as Rajwade, thirty-one out of thirty-eight officers in the WMS were Indian. Lady doctors left behind a legacy of enduring institutions that they founded. Muthulakshmi Reddy and Dr V. Shanta encouraged other women to do the same and lead, not follow. Post-independence India had its own successes. In 1947, Rajkumari Amrit Kaur, a protégé of Gandhi's, became the first health minister of independent India, serving in Jawaharlal Nehru's cabinet.

In Vellore, Dr Hilda Lazarus became the first Indian director of the famed Christian Medical College (CMC) in 1948. Lazarus was an evangelical Christian missionary, but she put religion to one side and made sure CMC provided healthcare to all. Sundara Ramachandran, the daughter of industrialist T.V. Sundaram Iyengar, was married at barely fourteen, but when her husband died, she went back to study at Lady Hardinge Medical College, graduating at the age of thirty-two in 1936. She joined the Gandhian movement, and in 1947, set up the Kasturba Hospital in Chinnalapatti, which focused on the welfare of women in rural areas.

The lady doctors also helped popularise Western medicine. Mary would fight a lone battle against homeopathy and for science. She valiantly defended vaccination programmes against homeopaths and quacks. The lady doctors battled for rationality and modern medicine against superstition.

Maternal health was revolutionised by women doctors. Muthulakshmi took part in civic sanitisation programmes. 'The pivot around which the improvement of maternal health revolved was the lady doctor,'[373] says medical historian and author Mridula Ramanna. Often, Indian women doctors would blend Eastern and Western methods, working with midwives rather than against them.

'Indian women physicians were indeed the vital intermediaries in promoting western medicine and disseminating knowledge about safer births, though this was mainly in the cities and towns,' adds Ramanna. 'They had the advantage of knowing the language, customs and the entrenched birthing practises.'[374]

Birth control was a controversial issue at the time. Muthulakshmi Reddy was firmly against it. Gandhian to the core, she thought it was 'unnatural' and instead advocated 'continence and self-control' along with late marriages. Luckily, others were more progressive, especially the Bombay physicians. Rajwade and Sukthankar both argued for birth control and the need to limit the population in a poor country with high infant mortality. Thanks to them, the AIWC adopted a resolution recommending that married men and women should be instructed in methods of birth control in recognised clinics. Muthulakshmi abstained from voting, but by 1940, enough medical support had built up that the Family Planning Society was set up. It would still take until 1952 for a nationwide family planning policy to come about, but the majority of women doctors supported planning.

Initially, the lady doctors were confined to helping women bear children, and many of them became ob-gyns. But by 1957, they had begun to practice general medicine, orthopaedics and other subjects. 'As in Britain, in India too, women were far keener to become doctors than to enter any other profession,' writes Ramanna. 'Besides, this was a space left to Indian women, where male doctors, both British and Indian, did not venture into, or even if they did, found women patients most reluctant to communicate their ailments to them.'[376]

Lastly, the respect that the lady doctors earned in their professions helped them move seamlessly into public life, and encouraged other women to be involved in public policy. Muthulakshmi helped to abolish the devadasi system, win women the vote and raise the age of marriage. Kadambini joined the Indian National Congress and was one of the first women to speak at their conferences. Rukhmabai, of course, defied an entire society to make it acceptable for Hindu women to divorce their husbands. Mary was the first Indian woman to be appointed to a legislature.

It is a cliché, but those who forget history are condemned to repeat it. The erasure of these early pioneers has resulted in an entire generation of Indians believing that women cannot excel in science. We rightly eulogise C.V. Raman and Jagdish Chandra Bose, but never the unsung women who fought far greater odds with unbelievable courage.

The lady doctors brought the beauty of science—its rigour, its certainty, its reassurance—to women who knew only superstition and chaos. Whether it was Rukhmabai fighting the plague, Haimabati delivering a baby or Muthulakshmi advocating for a cancer ward, they were fighting the dark shadows of ignorance. As we battle a global pandemic with vaccines that have been developed in record time, science is our only way out. When we talk about these lady doctors, we acknowledge the fight for knowledge and liberty. Let us keep their names alive.

Endnotes

1   Caroline Wells Healey Dall, *The Life of Dr Anandibai Joshi: A Kinswoman of the Pundita Ramabai* (Roberts Brothers, Boston, 1888), p. 48.

2   'Lady Surgeons', *British Medical Journal*, 2 April 1870, pp. 338–339.

3   Martha Vicinus and Bea Nergaard (eds.), *Ever Yours, Florence Nightingale: Selected Letters* (Harvard University Press, Boston, 1990), p. 210.

4   ibid.

5   David Kelly, 'Celebrated Ancient Egyptian Woman Physician Likely Never Existed, Says Researcher', University of Colorado press release, 18 December 2019.

6   Nicole Saldarriaga, 'Agnodice, the First Female Physician: Maybe', *Classical Wisdom*, 9 July 2015.

7   Irene Archos, 'Agnodice: The First Gyno to Greek Women', *Greek American Girl*, 1 March 2016.

8   Julia Boyd, 'Florence Nightingale's Remarkable Life and Work', *The Lancet*, 18 October 2008.

9   Michael Du Preez, 'Dr James Barry (1789–1865): The Edinburgh Years', *Journal of the Royal College of Physicians of Edinburgh*, 2012, vol. 42, pp. 258–265.

10   Lauren Young, 'Why This Groundbreaking British Doctor Was Almost Erased From the History Books', *Atlas Obscura*, 22 December 2016.

11   Alison Flood, 'New Novel about Dr James Barry Sparks Row over Victorian's Gender Identity', *The Guardian*, 18 February 2019.

12   Obituary of Elizabeth Blackwell, *The Lancet*, 6 November 1910.

13   Nancy Kline, *Elizabeth Blackwell: First Woman MD* (Conari Press, Berkeley, California, 1997), p. 56.

14   ibid., p. 61.

15   ibid., p. 60.

16   ibid., p. 74.

17   ibid., p. 83.

18   ibid., p. 84.

19   ibid., pp. 85–86.

20   ibid., p. 86.

21   ibid., p. 101.

22   Florence Nightingale, *Notes on Nursing* (D. Appleton and Co, New York, 1860), p. 52.

23   Elizabeth Garrett-Anderson, Inaugural Address delivered by Elizabeth Garret Anderson, H.K Lewis, London, 1877.

24   ibid., p. 14.

25   Margaret Georgina Todd, *The Life of Sophia Jex-Blake* (Macmillan, London, 1918), p. 32.

26   ibid., pp. 68–69.

27   ibid., p. 247.

28   ibid., p. 255.

29   ibid., p. 263.

30   ibid.

31   Sophia Jex-Blake, *Medical Women: A Thesis and a History* (Oliphant, Anderson and Ferrier, Edinburgh, 1886), pp. 92–93.

32   ibid., p. 104.

33   Simran Piya, 'Representing the Seven', https://blogs.ed.ac.uk/
edinburgh7/2019/07/04/representing-the-seven-simran-piya/.

34   ibid.

35   Malavika Karlekar, 'Elusive Voices: The Lives and Letters of
Anandibai Joshi', *Telegraph India*, 4 September 2007.

36   ibid.

37   Meera Kosambi, *A Fragmented Feminism: The Life and Letters
of Anandibai Joshi*, edited by Ram Ramaswamy, Madhavi Kolhatkar
and Aban Mukherjee (Taylor and Francis, New Delhi, 2019) p. 11.

38   Meera Kosambi, *Crossing Thresholds* (Permanent Black, New
Delhi, 2007), p. 174.

39   Kosambi, *A Fragmented Feminism*, p. 24.

40   ibid., p. 15.

41   Dall, *Anandibai Joshee*, p. 32.

42   Kosambi, *A Fragmented Feminism*, p. 25.

43   Dall, *Anandibai Joshee*, p. 30.

44   ibid., p. 34.

45   ibid., p. 40.

46   ibid., p. 52.

47   ibid., p. 52.

48   ibid., p. 72.

49   Dall, *Anandibai Joshee*, p. 82.

50   ibid.

51   ibid., pp. 83–86.

52   Kosambi, *A Fragmented Feminism*, p. 100.

53   Dall, *Anandibai Joshee*, p. 99.

54   ibid.

55   Kosambi, *A Fragmented Feminism*, p. 106.

56   ibid., p. 121.

57   ibid.

58   ibid.

59   Annika Burgess, 'Student Life at the First Medical College for Women', *Atlas Obscura*, 4 January 2018.

60   'Doctor or Doctress: Explore American History Through the Eyes of Women Physicians', Drexel University Legacy Centre, http://doctordoctress.org/islandora/object/islandora: 1496/story/islandora: 1541#page/44/mode/1up?width=1000&height=800&iframe=true>.

61   ibid.

62   Steven Jay, Peitzman *A New and Untried Course: Woman's Medical College and Medical College of Pennsylvania, 1850-1998* (Rutgers University Press, New Jersey, 2000), pp. 63–68.

63   ibid.

64   Burgess, 'Student Life', p. 1.

65   ibid.

66   ibid.

67   Sarah Pripas, 'The International History of Women's Medical Education', Nursing Clio, 16 June 2015.

68   Alissa Falcone, 'Remembering the Pioneering Women From One of Drexel's Legacy Medical Colleges', Drexel Now, 27 March 2017.

69   Kosambi, *A Fragmented Feminism*, p. 129.

70   ibid., p. 131.

71   ibid.

72   ibid., p. 154.

73   ibid., pp. 151–152.

74   ibid.

75   Dall, *Anandibai Joshee*, p. 109.

76   ibid., p. 11.

77   Kosambi, *A Fragmented Feminism*, p. 156.

78   Dall, *Anandibai Joshee*, p. 117.

79   Kosambi, *A Fragmented Feminism*, p. 138.

80   ibid.

81   ibid.

82   ibid., p. 142.

83   Dall, *Anandibai Joshee*, p. 131.

84   Kosambi, *A Fragmented Feminism*, p. 132.

85   ibid., p. 133.

86   ibid., p. 136.

87   Dall, *Anandibai Joshee*, p. 123.

88   Kosambi, *A Fragmented Feminism*, p. 200.

89   Dall, *Anandibai Joshee*, p. 142.

90   Kosambi, *A Fragmented Feminism*, pp. 200–202.

91   ibid.

92   ibid.

93   ibid., p. 144.

94   ibid., p. 145.

95   ibid., p. 185.

96   Kosambi, *A Fragmented Feminism*, p. 10.

97   Dall, p. 184.

98   ibid.

99   Kosambi, *A Fragmented Feminism*, p. 138.

100   Dall, *Anandibai Joshee*, p. 138.

101   Pushkar Sohani, 'A Controversy Over Tea', *Pune Mirror*, 2 September 2017.

102   Kosambi, *A Fragmented Feminism*, p. 236.

103   Ashim Kumar Dutta, 'The Brahmo Samaj and Women's Education in 19th Century Bengal', Bethune College Centenary Volume 1879-1979 (Calcutta, 1980), pp. 148–149.

104   S.N. Guha Ray, *Bethune School and College Centenary Volume 1849-1949* (Calcutta 1949).

105   Partha Sircar, 'Early Women's Education in Bengal and India', India Currents, 26 May 2016.

106   ibid.

107   Mousumi Bandyopadhyay, *Kadambini Ganguly: The Archetypal Woman of Nineteenth Century Bengal* (The Women's Press, London, 2011), p. 160.

108   ibid., p. 219.

109   ibid., p. 221.

110   David Kopf, *Brahmo Samaj and The Shaping of the Indian Mind* (Princeton Press, New Jersey, 1979), p. 125.

111   Email from Dr Mousumi Bandyopadhyay Majumdar, dated 19 March 2020.

112   ibid..

113   Bandyopadhyay, *Kadambini Ganguly*, p. 163.

114   B.K. Sen, 'Kadambini Ganguly: An Illustrious Lady', *Pune Mirror*, September–October 2014, p. 272.

115   Bandyopadhyay, *Kadambini Ganguly*, p. 209.

116   ibid., p. 210.

117   ibid., pp. 102–114.

118   Geraldine Forbes, 'Medical Careers and Health Care for Indian Women: Patterns of Control', *Women's History Review*, vol. 3, 4 November 1994.

119   Antoinette Burton, 'Contesting the Zenana: The Mission to Make Lady Doctors for India', *The Journal of British Studies*, vol. 35, no. 3, July 1996, pp. 368–397.

120   Bandyopadhyay, *Kadambini Ganguly*, p. 207.

121   Soma Basu, *Kadambini Ganguly: A Portrait of a Doctor at Dawn* (Rupali Press, New Delhi, 2012), p. 101.

122   Karlekar, *Kadambini and the Bhadralok*, vol. 21, no. 17 (26 April 1986), pp. WS25–WS31.

123   ibid.

124   Bandyopadhyay, *Kadambini Ganguly*, p. 209.

125   Mousumi Bandyopadhyay Majumdar, email of 19 March 2020.

126   Basu, *Kadambini Ganguly*, p. 81.

127   Bandyopadhyay, *Kadambini Ganguly*, p. 230.

128   ibid., p. 239.

129   Mohini Varde, *Dr Rakhmabai: An Odyssey* (New Delhi, Minerva Press, 2000), p. 61.

130   *The Times of India*, 9 April 1887.

131   ibid.

132   Sudhir Chandra, *Enslaved Daughters: Colonialism, Law and Women's Rights* (Oxford University Press, New Delhi 1998).

133   ibid.

134   *The Times of India*, 26 June 1885.

135   ibid.

136   ibid.

137   ibid.

138   Chandra, *Enslaved Daughters*.

139   *The Times of India*, 19 September 1885.

140   Varde, *Dr Rakhmabai: An Odyssey*, p. 64.

141   ibid.

142   Parimala V. Rao, *Foundations of Tilak's Nationalism: Discrimination, Education and Hindutva* (Orient Blackswan, New Delhi, 2010), p. 134.

143   'Higher Female Education', *The Mahratta*, 7 September 1884, cited by Parimala V. Rao, *Indian Historical Review*, vol. XXXV, no. 2, July 2008, pp. 155–177.

144   Rao, *Foundations of Tilak's Nationalism*, p. 105.

145   *The Mahratta*, 18 September 1887, cited by Parimala V. Rao, 'Women's Education and the Nationalist Response in Western India Part 1', *Indian Journal for Gender Studies*, 2007, p. 314.

146   *The Mahratta*, 5 July 1885, cited by Parimala V Rao, *Indian Historical Review*, pp. 155–177.

147   *The Mahratta*, 18 October 1885, ibid.

148   Rao, *Foundations of Tilak's Nationalism*, p. 97.

149   *Dadaji Bhikaji vs Rukhmabai* (1885) ILR 9 Bom 529.

150   ibid.

151   ibid.

152   *The Mahratta*, 11 October 1885.

153   *The Times of India*, 22 September 1885.

154   Chandra, *Enslaved Daughters*.

155   ibid.

156   ibid.

157   ibid.

158   ibid.

159   Stanley A. Wolpert, *Tilak and Gokhale: Revolution and Reform in the Making of Modern India* (University of California Press, Berkeley, 1962), pp. 35–42.

160   Parimala V. Rao, *Indian Historical Review*, p. 164.

161   *The Times*, 21 April 1887.

162   Chandra, *Enslaved Daughters*, p. 22.

163   ibid., p. 24.

164   Antoinette Burton, 'From Child Bride to Hindoo Lady: Rukhmabai and the Debate on Sexual Respectability in Imperial Britain', *The American Historical Review*, vol. 103, no. 4, October 1998, pp. 1119–1146.

165   ibid.

166   N.C Kelkar, *Life and Times of Lokmanya Tilak*, translated by D. Divekar (Radha Publications, Mumbai, 2001), p. 201.

167   Rao, *Nationalism and the Visibility of Women in Public Space*, p. 169.

168   ibid.

169   Wolpert, p. 297.

170   Varde, *Dr Rakhmabai: An Odyssey*, p. 100.

171   ibid., p. 105.

172   ibid., p. 108.

173   ibid.

174   ibid., p. 110.

175   ibid., p. 112.

176   Antoinette Burton, *The Heart of The Empire: Indians and the Colonial Encounter in Late Victorian Britain*, University of California Press, pp. 140–145.

177   ibid.

178   ibid.

179   ibid.

180   Cornelia Sorabji, *The Memories of Cornelia Sorabji* (Nisbet and Company, London, 1934) pp. 78–79.

181   ibid., p. 79.

182   Varde, *Dr Rakhmabai: An Odyssey*, p. 146.

183   Hannah Whitall Smith 'A Hindu Heroine', *The Woman's Signal Budget*, vol. 1, no. 3, November 1894, p. 21.

184   Varde, *Dr Rakhmabai: An Odyssey*, p. 128.

185   ibid., p. 133.

186   ibid.

187   ibid., pp. 130–131.

188   ibid., p. 134.

189   ibid., p. 153.

190   ibid., p. 156

191   ibid.

192   ibid., p. 158.

193   ibid., p. 196.

194   Haimabati Sen, *'Because I am a Woman': A Child Widow's Memoirs from Colonial India*, edited by Geraldine Forbes and Tapan Raychaudhuri (Chronicle Books, San Francisco, 2011), pp. 9–10.

195   ibid. p. 10.

196   ibid., p. 12.

197   ibid., p. 12.

198   ibid., p. 15.

199   ibid., p. 16.

200   ibid., p. 16.

201   Tapan Raychaudhuri, *Love in a Colonial Climate: Marriage, Romance and Sex in Nineteenth Century Bengal* (Cambridge University Press, Cambridge, 2000), pp. 349–378.

202   ibid.

203   ibid.

204   Haimabati Sen, *'Because I am a Woman'*, pp. 28–29.

205   ibid., p. 26.

206   ibid., p. 29.

207   ibid., p. 32.

208   ibid., p. 36.

209   ibid., p. 39.

210   ibid.

211   Teesta Setalvad, 'Anniversary Tribute: Think Hindu Widows' Remarriage, Think Vidyasagar', *Sabrang India*, 26 September 2016.

212   Ishwar Chandra Vidyasagar, *Hindu Widow Marriage*, translated by Brian. A. Hatcher, (Columbia University Press, New York, 2011), p. 70.

213   ibid.

214   Haimabati Sen, *'Because I am a Woman'*, p. 40.

215   ibid., p. 42.

216   E.B. Havell, *Benaras The Sacred City: Sketches of Hindu Life and Religion* (W. Thacker, 1911), p. 134.

217   Haimabati Sen, *'Because I am a Woman'*, p. 62.

218   ibid., p. 64.

219   ibid., p. 67.

220   ibid., p. 68.

221   ibid., p. 13.

222   ibid., p. 128.

223   ibid., p. 132.

224   Neha Banka, 'Streetwise Kolkata', *Indian Express*, 3 January 2020.

225   Geraldine Forbes, *Women in Colonial India* (DC Publishers, New Delhi, 2004), p. 123.

226   Geraldine Forbes, 'No Science for Lady Doctors', *Journal of the Asiatic Society of Bangladesh*, vol. 49, Issue 2, 2004, p. 271.

227   ibid., pp. 280–281.

228   Haimabati Sen, *'Because I am a Woman'*, p. 168.

229   ibid., p. 170.

230   ibid., p. 171.

231   ibid.

232   ibid., p. 174.

233   ibid., p. 176.

234   ibid., p. 175.

235   ibid.

236   ibid., p. 181..

237   ibid., p. 184.

238   ibid.

239   ibid., p. 189.

240   ibid., p. 191.

241   ibid., p. 193.

242   ibid., p. 195.

243   ibid., p. 210.

244   Geraldine Forbes, *Women in Colonial India*, p. 121.

245   ibid., p. 130.

246   Haimabati Sen, *'Because I am a Woman'*, p. 227.

247   ibid., p. 231.

248   ibid.

249   ibid., p. 239.

250   Indrani Sen, 'Resisting Patriarchy: Complexities and Conflicts in the Memoir of Haimabati Sen,' *Economic & Political Weekly*, vol. 47, no. 12, 24 March 2012.

251   ibid.

252   Haimabati Sen, *'Because I am a Woman'*, p. 242.

253   Muthulakshmi Reddy, *My Experience as a Legislator* (Current Thought Press, Chennai, 1930), p. 6.

254   ibid.

255   Muthulakshmi Reddy, *Autobiography* (Chennai, 1964), p. 7.

256   Aparna Basu, *The Pathfinder: Dr Muthulakshmi Reddy* (AIWC, New Delhi, 1987), p. 3.

257   *Pudukottai Gazetteer*, 1904.

258   V. Shanta , 'A Legend Unto Herself' (India International Centre, New Delhi, Occasional no 44).

259   Muthulakshmi Reddy, *Autobiography*, p. 4.

260   ibid., p. 4.

261   ibid., p. 5.

262   ibid., p. 7.

263   ibid., p. 7.

264   S. Mutthiah, *Madras Musings*, 15 April 2008.

265   Muthulakshmi Reddy, *Autobiography*, p. 11.

266   The National Medical Journal of India (vol. 23:2, 2010), p. 118.

267   S. Muthiah, 'Madras Miscellany', *The Hindu*, 6 October 2013.

268   Muthulakshmi Reddy, *Autobiography*, p. 13.

269   ibid.

270   S. Muthiah, 'Madras Miscellany', *The Hindu*, 18 March 2019.

271   Muthulakshmi Reddy, *Autobiography*, p. 11.

272   ibid., p. 18.

273   ibid., p. 22.

274   ibid., p. 23.

275   ibid., p. 22.

276   ibid., p. 35.

277   ibid., p. 36.

278   ibid.

279   ibid., p. 42.

280   ibid.

281   'The Lyrics: A Casket of Vocal Gems from the Golden Age of Music Hall', Monologues.co.uk.

282   Geraldine Forbes, *Women in Colonial India*, p. 66.

283   Menon, Nitya 'When Chennai's Women Won the Vote', *The Hindu*, 8 March 2015.

284   ibid., p. 100.

285   Geraldine Forbes, *Women in Colonial India*, p. 76.

286   ibid.

287   Muthulakshmi Reddy, *My Experiences as a Legislator*, p. 1.

288   *The Hindu* (Editorial), 15 August 1947.

289   Muthulakshmi Reddy, *Autobiography*, p. 105.

290   Interview with Dr V. Shanta in Chennai, 6 March 2020.

291   Kay Jordan, *From Sacred Servant to Profane Prostitute, a history of the changing legal status of the devadasis of India, 1857-1947* (Manohar Publishers and Distributors, Delhi, 2003)), p. 21.

292   Rao Sahib Abrahama M. Pandither, *Karunamirtha Sagaram, Book 1* (*Karunanithi Medical Hall*, Tanjore, 1970), p. 18.

293   J.A Dubois, *Hindu Manners, Customs and Ceremonies* (Clarendon Press, Oxford, 1897) p. 596.

294   V. Sriram, *The Devadasi and the Saint: The life and times of Bangalore Nagarathnamma* (East West, Chennai 2016).

295   ibid.

296   ibid.

297   ibid.

298   Ranjani Govind, 'The Activist Behind the Music', *The Hindu*, 8 January 2016.

299   Muthulakshmi Reddy, *Autobiography*, p. 67.

300   ibid., p. 68.

301   Sriram, *The Devadasi and the Saint*.

302   ibid.

303   ibid.

304   Muthulakshmi Reddy, *My Experiences as a Legislator*, p. 154.

305   Muthulakshmi Reddy, *My Experiences as a Legislator*, p. 101.

306   ibid.

307   ibid.

308   ibid., p. 107.

309   Muthulakshmi Reddy, *Autobiography*, p. 59.

310   Avvai Home website.

311   S. Krishnamurthi, *Five Decades of the Cancer Institute (WIA): 1954-2004*, (Adyar Cancer Institute, Chennai, 1995), p. 22.

312   Kamala Ganesh, 'Dr Muthulakshmi Reddy, A Powerful face of Nationalist Feminism', *The Wire*, 1 August 2019.

313   Interview with Dr V. Shanta in Chennai, 6 March 2020.

314   Krishnamurthi, *Five Decades of the Cancer Institute*, p. 17.

315   Dr V. Shanta, Home page of Adyar Cancer Hospital.

316   Dr V. Shanta, Memory oration of Dr V. Krishnamurthi, http://cancerinstitutewia.in/CIWIA/dr_sk.html.

317   Cancer Institute WIA (Adyar) web page. cancerinstitutewia.in.

318   Krishnamurthi, *Five Decades of the Cancer Institute*, p. 30.

319   Interview with Dr Shanta, 6 March 2020, Chennai.

320   Dr V. Shanta, Memory oration of Dr V Krishnamurthi, http://cancerinstitutewia.in/CIWIA/dr_sk.html.

321   Interview with Dr V. Shanta in Chennai, 6 March 2020.

322   Interview with Dr V. Shanta, 6 March 2020, Chennai.

323   Dr V. Shanta, Muthulakshmi Reddy: A Legend unto Herself, p. 13

324   Dr V. Shanta, Memory oration of Dr V. Krishnamurthi, http://cancerinstitutewia.in/CIWIA/dr_sk.html.

325   Arundhati Roy, The God of Small Things (Penguin Random House, New Delhi, 2008), p. 3.

326   Robin Jeffrey, The Decline of Nayar Dominance: Society and Politics in Travancore, 1847-1908 (Vikas Publishing House, New Delhi, 1976), p. 19.

327   ibid., p. 18.

328   Mary Poonen Lukose, Trailblazer: The Legendary Life and Times of Mary Poonen Lukose, Surgeon General of Travancore, compiled by Leena Chandran (Malayala Manorama, Kottayam, 2019), p. 22.

329   Manu Pillai, 'The Good Doctor of Travancore', Mint, 8 August 2019.

330   Lukose, p. 26

331   ibid.

332   Lukose, p. 30.

333   ibid., p. 98.

334   Ramachandra Guha, 'How the Suffragettes influenced Mahatma Gandhi', Hindustan Times, 24 February 2018.

335   Steve Smith and Julie Smith, A Fiercely Independent Woman (Moonbrand Publications, London, 2013), p. 32.

336   Lukose, p. 104.

337   D. Stevens, 'Pride, Prejudice and Paediatrics', Archives of Disease in Childhood, 91(12), 2006, p. 1047.

338   ibid.

339   'Everywoman in 1910: No Vote, Poor Pay, Little Help—Why the World had to Change', Daily Mirror, 8 March 2010.

340   ibid.

341   Lukose, p. 40.

342   ibid., p. 39.

343   ibid., p. 34.

344   ibid., p. 37.

345   ibid., p. 43.

346   ibid., p. 56.

347   ibid., p. 52.

348   ibid.

349   ibid., p. 57.

350   ibid., p. 57.

351   ibid., p. 126.

352   Lukose, p. 96.

353   Francis Younghusband, *The Epic of Mount Everest* (Pan Macmillan, London 2000), p. 74.

354   Ed Douglas 'My Modest Father Never Mentioned His Everest Expedition Olympic Gold', *The Guardian*, 19 May 2012.

355   Theodore Howard Somervell, *Knife and Life in India: Being the Story of a Surgical Missionary at Neyvoor*, Travancore (Livingstone Press, London, 1940), p. 33.

356   ibid., p. 34.

357   ibid., pp. 97–98.

358   Manu Pillai, *Ivory Throne: Chronicles of the House of Travancore* (HarperCollins, New Delhi, 2015), p. 45.

359   ibid., p. 46.

360   Pillai, *The Ivory Throne*, p. 345.

361   ibid., p. 346.

362   Lukose, *Trailblazer*, p. 88.

363   ibid., p. 122.

364   Robin Jeffrey, *Politics, Women and Well Being: How Kerala became a Model* (Macmillan, New Delhi, 1992), pp. 94–95.

365   Travancore Legislative Assembly Proceedings, vol. 12, p. 125.

366   ibid., p. 132.

367   ibid.

368   ibid., p. 134.

369   ibid., p. 142.

370   ibid., p. 144.

371   Lukose, *Trailblazer*, p. 74.

372   'Kerala Budget 2018, Remembering an Extraordinary Talent of Mary Poonen Lukose', *Indian Express*, 2 February 2018.

373   Mridula Ramanna, *Health Care in the Bombay Presidency: 1896-1930* (Primus Books, New Delhi), p. 139.

374   ibid., p. 154.

Bibliography

Books

Antoinette Burton, *The Heart of The Empire: Indians and the Colonial Encounter in Late Victorian Britain*, University of California Press, Berkeley, 1998.

Aparna Basu, *The Pathfinder: Dr Muthulakshmi Reddy*, AIWC, New Delhi, 1987.

Arundhati Roy, *The God of Small Things*, Penguin Random House, New Delhi, 2008.

Caroline Wells Healey Dall, *The Life of Dr Anandabai Joshee: A Kinswoman of the Pundita Ramabai*, Roberts Brothers, Boston, 1888.

Cornelia Sorabji, *The Memories of Cornelia Sorabji*, Nisbet and Company, London, 1934.

David Kopf, *Brahmo Samaj and the Shaping of the Indian Mind*, Princeton Press, New Jersey, 1979.

Florence Nightingale, *Notes on Nursing*, D. Appleton and Co, New York, 1860.

Florence Nightingale, *Selected Letters*, Harvard University Press, Boston, 1990.

Geraldine Forbes, *Women in Colonial India*, DC Publishers, New Delhi, 2004.

Haimabati Sen, *Because I am a Woman: A Child Widow's Memoirs from Colonial India*, edited by Geraldine Forbes and Tapan Raychaudhuri, Chronicle Books, San Francisco, 2011.

Ishwar Chandra Vidyasagar, *Hindu Widow Marriage*, translated by Brian Hatcher, Columbia University Press, New York, 2011.

J.A. Dubois, *Hindu Manners, Customs and Ceremonies*, Clarendon Press, Oxford, 1897.

Kay Jordan, *From Sacred Servant to Profane Prostitute, a History of the Changing Legal Status of the Devadasis of India*, 1857–1947, Manohar Publishers and Distributors, Delhi, 2003.

Manu Pillai, *Ivory Throne: Chronicles of the House of Travancore*, HarperCollins, New Delhi, 2015.

Margaret Todd, *The Life of Sophia Jex-Blake*, Macmillan, London, 1918.

Martha Vicinus and Bea Nergaard (eds), Ever Yours', Florence Nightingale: Selected Letters, Harvard University Press, Boston, 1990.

Meera Kosambi, *A Fragmented Feminism: The Life and Letters of Anandibai Joshi*, edited by Ram Ramaswamy, Madhavi Kolhatkar and Aban Mukherjee, Taylor and Francis, New Delhi, 2019.

Mohini Varde, *Dr Rakhmabai: An Odyssey*, Minerva Press, New Delhi, 2000.

Mousumi Bandyopadhyay, *Kadambini Ganguly: The Archetypal Woman of Nineteenth Century Bengal*, The Women Press, New Delhi, 2011.

Mridula Ramanna, *Health Care in the Bombay Presidency: 1896–1930*, Primus Books, New Delhi.

Muthulakshmi Reddy, *My Autobiography*, Chennai, 1964.

Muthulakshmi Reddy, *My Experience as a Legislator*, Current Thought Press, Chennai, 1930.

N.C. Kelkar, *Life and Times of Lokmanya Tilak*, translated by D. Divekar. Radha Publications, Mumbai, 2001.

Nancy Kline, *Elizabeth Blackwell: First Woman M.D.*, Conari Press, Berkeley, California, 1997.

Parimala V. Rao, *Foundations of Tilak's Nationalism: Discrimination, Education and Hindutva*, Orient Blackswan, New Delhi, 2010.

Bibliography

Robin Jeffrey, *The Decline of Nayar Dominance: Society and Politics in Travancore, 1847–1908*, Vikas Publishing House, New Delhi, 1976.

S. Krishnamurthi, *Five Decades of the Cancer Institute*, WIA Institute, Chennai, 2004.

Soma Basu, *Kadambini Ganguly: A Portrait of a Doctor at Dawn*, Rupali Press, New Delhi, 2012.

Sophia Jex-Blake, *Medical Women: A Thesis and a History*, Oliphant, Anderson and Ferrier, Edinburgh, 1886.

Stanley A. Wolpert, *Tilak and Gokhale: Revolution and Reform in the Making of Modern India*, University of California Press, Berkeley, 1962.

Steve and Julie Smith, *A Fiercely Independent Woman*, Moonbrand Publications, London, 2013.

Sudhir Chandra, *Enslaved Daughters: Colonialism, Law and Women's Rights*, Oxford University Press, New Delhi, 1998.

Tapan Raychaudhuri, *Love in a Colonial Climate: Marriage, Romance and Sex in Nineteenth Century Bengal*, Cambridge University Press, Cambridge, 2000.

Theodore Howard Somervell, *Knife and Life in India: Being the Story of a Surgical Missionary at Neyyoor, Travancore*, Livingstone Press, London, 1940.

Trailblazer: The Legendary Life and Times of Dr Mary Poonen Lukose, Surgeon General of Travancore, Malayala Manorama, Kottayam, 2019.

V. Sriram, *The Devadasi and the Saint: The Life and Times of Bangalore Nagarathnamma*, East West, Chennai, 2016.

Articles

Alison Flood, 'New Novel about Dr James Barry Sparks Row over Victorian's Gender Identity', The Guardian, 18 February 2019.

Alissa Falcone, 'Remembering the Pioneering Women from One of Drexel's Legacy Medical Colleges', Drexel Now, 27 March 2017.

Annika Burgess, 'Student Life at the First Medical College for Women', Atlas Obscura, 4 January 2018.

Antoinette Burton, 'Contesting the Zenana: The Mission to Make Lady Doctors for India', t, vol. 35, no. 3, July 1996.

Ashim Kumar Dutta, 'The Brahmo Samaj and Women's Education in 19th Century Bengal', Bethune College Centenary Volume 1879-1979, 1980.

K. Sen, 'Kadambini Ganguly: An Illustrious Lady', Pune Mirror, September–October 2014.

David Kelly, 'Celebrated Ancient Egyptian Woman Physician Likely Never Existed, Says Researcher', University of Colorado press release, 18 December 2019.

Geraldine Forbes, 'No Science for Lady Doctors', Journal of the Asiatic Society of Bangladesh, vol. 49, issue 2, 2004.

Geraldine Forbes, 'Medical Careers and Health Care for Indian Women: Patterns of Control', Women's History Review, vol. 3, 4 November 1994.

Indrani Sen, 'Resisting Patriarchy: Complexities and Conflicts in the Memoir of Haimabati Sen', Economic amd Political Weekly, vol. 47, no. 12, 24 March 2012.

Irene Archos, 'Agnodice: The First Gyno to Greek Women', Greek American Girl, 1 March 2016.

Julia Boyd, 'Florence Nightingale's Remarkable Life and Work', The Lancet, 18 October 2008.

June Purvis, 'Everywoman in 1910: No Vote, Poor Pay, Little Help— Why the World Had to Change', Daily Mirror, 8 March 2010.

Kamala Ganesh, 'Dr Muthulakshmi Reddy, A Powerful face of

Nationalist Feminism', The Wire, 1 August 2019.

'Kerala Budget 2018: Remembering an Extraordinary Talent of Mary Poonen Lukose', New Indian Express, 2 February 2018.

'Lady Surgeons', British Medical Journal, 2 April 1870.

Lauren Young, 'Why This Ground-breaking British Doctor Was Almost Erased From the History Books', Atlas Obscura, 22 December 2016.

Malavika Karlekar, 'Elusive Voices: The Lives and Letters of Anandibai Joshi', Telegraph India, 4 September 2007.

Malavika Karlekar, 'Kadambini and the Bhadralok', Economic and Political Weekly, vol. 21, no. 17, 26 April 1986.

Michael Du Preez, 'Dr James Barry (1789–1865): The Edinburgh Years', Journal of the Royal College of Physicians of Edinburgh, 2012, vol. 42.

Nicole Saldarriaga, 'Agnodice, the First Female Physician: Maybe', Classical Wisdom, 9 July 2015.

Nitya Menon, 'When Chennai's Women Won the Vote', The Hindu, 8 March 2015.

Parimala Rao, 'Women's Education and the Nationalist Response in Western India Part 1', Indian Journal for Gender Studies, 2007.

Pushkar Sohani, 'A Controversy Over Tea', Pune Mirror, 2 September 2017.

Ramachandra Guha, 'How the Suffragettes influenced Mahatma Gandhi', Hindustan Times, 24 February 2018.

Ranjani Govind, 'The Activist Behind the Music,' The Hindu, 8 January 2016.

S. Muthiah, 'Madras Miscellany', The Hindu, 6 October 2013.

S.N. Guha Ray, Bethune School and College Centenary Volume 1849– 1949, 1949.

Travancore Legislative Assembly Proceedings, vol. 12.

Acknowledgements

This book grew from a Google Doodle. I saw the doodle celebrating Rukhmabai Raut, and was curious enough to read more about her. Her story led me down the fascinating rabbit hole of early women doctors. I was aided in this quest by many:

My steadfast friend and agent, Jayapriya Vasudevan of the Jacaranda Literary Agency, who saw the potential in what was only a half-formed idea, and helped me develop it into a book.

My writing group, who gave me absolutely invaluable feedback and put up with my incessant moaning: Madhumita, Monika, Radhika, Rohini, Shruthi, Sonya, Sushmita (alphabetical order), this book belongs to you as much as to me.

My wonderful editor Deepthi Talwar, who whipped this long and meandering book into shape as only she can.

Dr V. Shanta, an icon who sadly passed away before she could see this book, but gave me so much of her scarce time.

Dr Mohini Varde and Dr Mousumi Bandyopadhyay Majumdar, who helped me a great deal with their anecdotes and recollections.

Dr Geraldine Forbes, who kindly sent me copies of her books and advised on the subject.

Leena Chandran and Kuruvilla Lukose, who were generous with contacts and photos.

Agnes Kindrachuk, who went out of her way to help me with the research.

Raina Assainar and Geetha Srimathi, who helped me with translation and photo sourcing.

My cat Idli, who got me through the toughest bits of this book with his purring and cuddles.

Most importantly: my mother, who stood firm by me through the writing of this book during a pandemic, as she has always stood by me through life.

About the Author

Kavitha Rao is a London-based author and journalist. Her work has appeared in the *Guardian*, *New York Times*, *South China Morning Post*, Mint, *The Hindu* and various others. *Lady Doctors* is her third book. She is on Twitter at @kavitharao.